THE
SCIATICA
RELIEF
HANDBOOK

By CHET CUNNINGHAM

With a foreword by:
Dr. Mary Ann Castor
D.C., R.N.

UNITED RESEARCH PUBLISHERS

CONTENTS

i

Contents

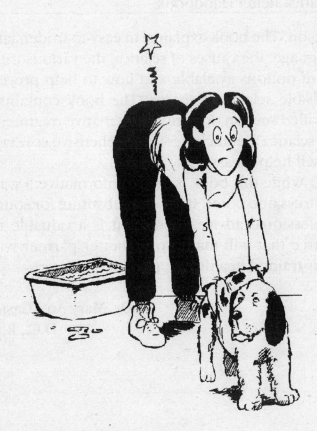

FOREWORD

Thousands of Americans suffer from sciatica, yet information on this subject is scarce. I visited several local bookstores and could not find a single book on the subject of sciatica.

That's why this book is of vital importance—it fills a much-needed information void for the lay person. The book explains, in easy-to-understand language, the causes of sciatica, the various treatment options available and how to help prevent possible sciatica flare-ups. The book contains a detailed section on various alternative treatments for sciatica and includes comprehensive coverage of self-help measures.

While this book is highly informative, I want to stress one point: It is not a substitute for sound professional advice. Instead, it is a valuable resource that will make you a better partner with your trained health care provider.

Dr. Mary Ann Castor
D.C., R.N.

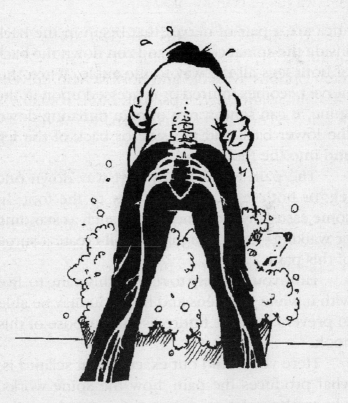

INTRODUCTION

◆ Sometimes it hurts so bad you want to scream.
◆ It's a pain down the back of one or both legs
  that gives you fits.
◆ It hurts like fire whenever you move.
◆ What is it and how can you get rid of it?

We're talking about sciatica pain here. The sci-

3

atica are a pair of nerves that begin in the back inside the spinal column and run down the back of both legs all the way to the ankle. When this nerve becomes injured or is pressed upon in the spine, it can send waves of pain radiating down the lower back and the side or back of the leg and into the foot.

The pain may be only part way down one leg, or both legs, or all the way to the foot. In some cases any movement at all such as standing or walking—even coughing—will create a surge of this pain.

How you can help to reduce this pain, to live with it while it lessens and how you may be able to prevent it in the future, is the purpose of this book.

Here you'll find out exactly what sciatica is, what produces the pain, how the spine works, where the sciatica pain originates, how the spine's injury or wear and tear can produce the pain, and how sciatica can be treated with everything from diet and acupuncture to medications and in the ultimate extreme, surgery.

While sciatica pain may have any one of several causes, it usually is a direct result of an injury to or wear and tear of the discs that separate your spine's vertebrae. These discs act as shock absorbers and separators and let your spine and

4

your back twist and turn and move without any pain. That's a normal disc.

The disc itself is made up of a soft inner core and a harder, tougher outer covering. Think about a donut with a jelly filled center; that's like a disc in your spine.

Sciatica pain comes when one of the discs prolapses. This is when the soft pulpy core of the disc bulges out or is pushed out through the outer covering and presses against the sciatic nerve which runs down the spine.

This book will go into detail about how this happens and when it does what you can do yourself to help relieve the pain. We'll show the various methods of treating sciatica, some that work and some that are little more than hype and wishful thinking and "cash cows" for the proponents.

Sciatica is often the direct result of bad back management, poor posture and years of misuse of your back through lifting objects the wrong way, bad sitting and standing posture and even the wrong way lying down. Since the whole back affects the spine and the discs, we'll show you the proper way to take care of your back so you'll have less chance of a sciatica attack. If you do have sciatica, this book will help you learn more about the problem, and then show you how you can do a lot of self treatment and how to get the best medical care for your problem.

Yes, exercises are a vital part of a healthy back. To this end there are a number of exercises detailed here that show you how to take care of your back, and how to strengthen the back and stomach muscles to help you prevent that dreaded low back pain and how to lessen your chances of any more sciatica attacks.

You may have heard that back pains are one of the largest causes of visits to a doctor's office. Probably true. You may also have heard that for those with bad back pain, half can be successfully treated by a medical doctor, half can be successfully treated with physical therapy or a chiropractor, and that the other half can find relief by doing absolutely nothing and let nature do the healing. All three "cures" for sciatica work about the same. The two former ones will help reduce the time frame of your pain and are the usual treatment of choice by most victims of back pain.

So, where does that leave you, the average back pain person who has had or may have sciatica? By reading and putting into practice the suggestions here, you will be in the proverbial driver's seat, with the knowledge and understanding you need to treat your sciatica and your back the most efficient and pain relieving way. It helps you know when to go see your doctor. It

6

also helps you to prevent back pain in the future by taking better care of your back, and setting up an exercise program to strengthen your whole back, which will help reduce the chance of a sciatica attack.

What's next? Charge into Chapter One and find out all there is to know about sciatica.

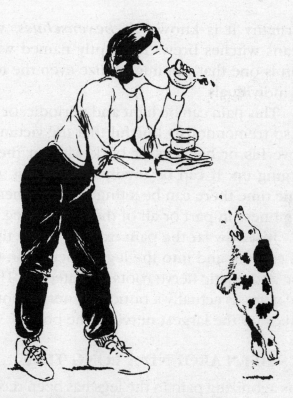

CHAPTER ONE:
WHAT IS SCIATICA?

Sciatica is a condition of the spinal column where some object is pressing against the sciatic nerve root which results in serious pain in the lower back and buttocks often radiating down one or both legs, sometimes all the way into the foot. In

Germany it is known as *hexenschuss*, which means witches brew. This aptly named witches pain is one that can immobilize even the toughest individuals.

This pain can be light and periodic, or it can be so tremendously hurtful that the victim can't move his or her legs or back without the pain surging up. It can be totally debilitating. At the same time there can be a tingling, weakness and numbness in part or all of the affected leg.

Just how far the pain extends down the spinal column and into the legs depends on which disc and sciatic nerve roots are affected. The sciatic nerve is actually a bundle of nerve roots and makes up the largest nerve in the body.

IT'S BEEN AROUND A LONG TIME

This agonizing pain in the legs has been recorded in history down through the ages. Hippocrites, the Greek physician, in the fifth century B.C. wrote that Scythians had a lot of sciatica pain which he attributed to their riding so much on horses.

Roman Pliny the Elder noted five hundred years later that he had a cure for this sciatica pain. It was called hiberis and was made from earthworm washings.

Shakespeare in seventeenth century England

used the term in one of his plays when Timon of Athens said: "Thou cold sciatica, cripple our senators."

Doctors laid the cause of sciatica to a great many reasons, all which proved to be wrong until in the l930's when two doctors discovered that sciatica often was caused by the herniation of one or more intervertebral discs.

WHY DO DISCS BULGE AND RUPTURE?

Those intervertebral discs are the villains. What are they? Between your vertebrae are twenty-three discs that serve as cushions to let your spine do the work it must do. These discs are made up of a wet, spongy inner core and a stiff, sturdier outer shell that keeps the disc intact.

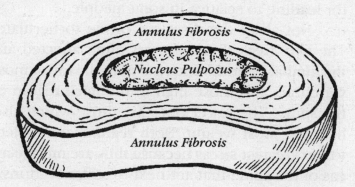

After a person is twenty years old, these discs

begin to wear in relation to the amount of pressure and movement the spine is subjected to. Many people have sciatic pain in the late twenties. It becomes more prevalent in people from thirty to fifty years of age. The age of thirty-eight is average for patients having lumbar disc surgery.

While age often is a factor, that isn't the cause of sciatica. There are a complex group of other factors that have a bearing. These include work that requires repetitive lifting, constant exposure to vibrations like long rides on a motorcycle or driving a car or truck for long periods of time. Dr. John Frymoyer in an article in *The New England Journal of Medicine* said that there may also be a correlation between sciatica pain and job dissatisfaction and depression. Another study showed that cigarette smoking could be a risk factor leading to sciatica in some people.

Not all of the discs are prone to herniate. The two areas that are most often affected are the lumbar region, which includes the lower most vertebrae, and those high in the neck region of the spine. The lower ones are those which also bear the most weight. Both regions are subject to the greatest stress because they are mobile areas of the spine that are next to stiffer sections.

If the disc that herniates is in the neck region, it will produce pain in the neck and radiat-

Cross-section View

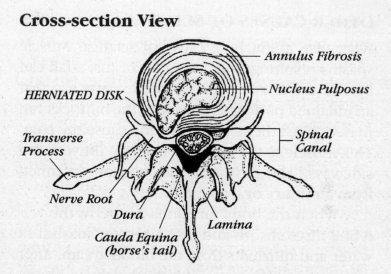

ing out into the arms sometimes and all the way into the hands, resulting in numbness and muscle weakness. If the protrusion from a bulging or herniated disc touches nerve roots in the cauda equina, the patient may have trouble urinating or defecating. These are the nerves that control the bowels and bladder. Most sciatica problems deal with pain in the buttocks and down the legs to the feet.

When a disc herniates it is almost always the final phase of a long process of wear and tear on the disc caused by work habits, or lifting or straining. The final "blow out" of the disc might come from some innocent movement such as picking up a newspaper or bending over to sit down.

OTHER CAUSES OF SCIATICA

What else might be a cause of sciatica? Muscle spasms resulting from an injury or just a fall can irritate the sciatic nerve. Some experts say that an inflamed piriformis muscle in the buttocks can press against the sciatic nerve and cause the pain. This muscle is the one that lets you lift your leg sideways. The piriformis can become inflamed from an injury or over-exertion.

When the body functions properly, the vertebral discs absorb and lose a certain amount of water and nutrients from the bloodstream. After a person is thirty years old, this balanced operation goes a little out of whack, and the discs begin to lose a little more water than they absorb. So the disc begins to dry out. This causes the width of the disc to shrink. Over the next thirty to forty years, each disc may lose up to one eighth of an inch in thickness. Multiply this times twenty-three and you see why your grandmother is shorter now then she used to be by three or four inches.

The drying out has other problems as well. If the outer layer dries out quicker than the soft inner layer, it can often result in a "leak" or rupture in the outer layer. When a leak occurs the soft inner core of the disc drains through the outer layer. When this happens the protrusion

14

often presses against the sciatica nerve root. This pressure produces the pains and discomforts of sciatica.

If the outer shell isn't broken but is bulged out by the pressure of the inner layer, the same thing can happen. The bulge of the harder layer presses against the sciatic nerve and triggers the pain.

This condition almost always happens in one of the lower lumbar discs. This rupture of the disc can take place and not cause any pain, as long as the material does not press against or interfere with the work of the sciatic nerve roots. Such sciatic pain happens to about ten percent of the population.

Richard W. Porter, MD, says that only about ten percent of patients with a disc protrusion actually develop any pain from them.
He says in the other ninety percent the spinal canal is usually wide enough for the nerve to escape any damage from the bulging disc. Dr. Porter is a professor of orthopaedics at the University of Aberdeen in Scotland.

Dr. Porter says that inflammatory mediators from the nucleus of the disc that may be touching the nerves may also be responsible for some of the sciatica pain.

NO SUCH THING AS A SLIPPED DISC

This herniated disc condition is often referred to by the public as a "slipped disc" which is incorrect. There is no slippage whatsoever of the affected disc. Old labels die hard, and this condition probably will be called by this name for many years yet.

In some cases this bit of material that oozes out of the disc can become disconnected from the rest of the core material. Doctors then say that it is "sequestered" since it is alone. It may remain in the spinal canal and cause further problems or it may remain in place and not cause any trouble.

Usually the material from the disc core remains attached and the body starts the healing process of repairing the "leak" or bulge in the outer shell.

With the bulging disc the protrusion may not press on the nerve so much that it "pinches" it and causes it to malfunction. Many times the bulging is minor and simply irritates the nerve roots, but still causes severe pain.

Most sciatica pain is in the buttocks and legs, because of the way the nerve bundles are located. Sometimes nerves are affected which extend into the back and this will produce sciatic pain in the back as well as the lower extremities.

Such a bulging disc might cause you pain three or four times a year, and when it shrinks down the pain then goes away. These bulges might come for a variety of reasons including simple motions like bending forward. This can put a strain on the lower discs and cause a problem if the rear wall of the disc is weakened.

POSTURE IS STRESSFUL ON THOSE LUMBAR DISCS

A Swedish orthopaedic surgeon, Dr. Alf Nachemson, made a study of which postures and positions put the most strain on the lumbar spine discs. He found that lying on your back is least stressful with a rating of twenty-five. Lying on your side is three times as stressful, and the act of standing produces a rating of one hundred. Standing and bending over and lifting an item is more stressful with a rating of two hundred and twenty-five. Sitting and bending to the floor to pick up an object is the most stressful with a total of two hundred and seventy-five.

Curiously, sitting down is more stressful at one hundred and forty than standing is at one hundred points.

From long experience, doctors have found that a minor bulging of a disc will usually vanish along with the pain after a good night's rest. On the other extreme, some bulging discs may take three or four months to heal and for the pain to go away. Doctors say that even the most severely herniated disc should heal after nine months. Most sciatic pain should be gone after sixty days.

MORE CAUSES OF SCIATICA PAIN

The disc is the major cause of sciatica pain, but it can also be triggered by infections, injuries, tumors, arthritis, ankylosing spondyltis, a condition known as spondylolisthesis and spinal stenosis. Let's check out some of these.

Arthritis

There are three types of arthritis that affect the spine: degenerative arthritis, osteoarthritis and rheumatoid arthritis.

Degenerative arthritis is by far the most common and at the same time usually the least serious. This is a normal part of the aging process. This simply means that as we get older, the more our joints wear and some of them wear out. The problem is that the cartilage that cushions and protects the joints wears away. The joints most affected include the hands and feet and the spine.

When the cartilage wears thin and the discs

shrink down because of age and wear and tear, there's more chance of the sciatica nerve roots in the spinal canal being affected.

Osteoarthritis is the growing of rims or bony spurs either on or near the facet joints. They actually help stabilize the discs or joints of the spine and may help avoid back pain, not cause it. In people over sixty-five this condition may limit mobility and cause some stiffness of the back. However osteoarthritis is not a big factor in back pain and rarely is there any serious problem involved.

Rheumatoid arthritis can attack the spinal column, but it also is a body wide disease affecting the joints in the hands, elbows, fingers, toes and shoulders as well. If it affects the facet joints of the spine, it results in severe inflammation, swelling and painful stiffness. Rheumatoid arthritis can destroy the joint as it progresses as well as the tissue surrounding it.

Ankylosing Spondylitis

This is a severe inflammation of the spinal joints that then stiffen and causes severe pain. It usually starts at the base of the spine and works its way upward. Twice as many men are affected as women and it usually starts in the late twenties. As it progresses, the vertebrae fuse and the victim hunches over until he can hardly see ahead. This is another of the diseases of the spine we're not concerned with here.

Spondylolisthesis

Spondylolisthesis is the real slipped disc. For this to happen, first there must be a crack in the back of a vertebra. When this crack widens sufficiently, the front section of the vertebra can then slip forward in relation to the vertebra below it. In a mild form this problem can go unnoticed since there is little or no pain involved. A flare up of pain may come from sudden exertion. The best treatment is exercises to strengthen the area after the pain subsides.

Spinal Stenosis

Another way that sciatica pain can develop is from spinal stenosis. This means narrowing and here applies to the narrowing of the spinal canal through which the sciatica nerve passes.

This problem comes with the advent of degenerative arthritis when the formation of bone spurs on the spine can change the contours of the vertebrae.

There are a wide variety of ways that this narrowing affects the sciatic nerve depending where the narrowing takes place. It can mean the tingling, numbness and the shooting pain and weakness usually associated with sciatica.

DIAGNOSING IT

When you have a serious back pain and go to your doctor, he will start by taking a history of your back problem. Doctors tell us that it is difficult to diagnose a bulging disc quickly. He will start by asking you several questions. He'll ask if you've had any work where you had to do a lot of lifting or if you've had any recent falls or injury to your back or legs. Most doctors agree that back pains are hard to diagnose.

The diagnosis of pains in the back that the doctor thinks may come from a ruptured disc is sometimes helped by reading the patient's symptoms. If the sudden pain is "electric" and results in a burning sensation and sometimes numbing and tingling, it usually is determined to be sciatica and not the milder buttocks and leg pain from a facet joint problem. The facet joint is what holds the vertebrae together.

Sciatica pain usually is more severe when bending forward and when coughing or sneezing and this is another way to help diagnose it.

By flexing the neck forward increased stress is placed on the spinal cord. If there is a herniated disc, such neck flexing can create a sharp

21

pain down the legs or in the buttocks, and sciatica is the diagnosis.

A physical examination should be a part of every doctor's evaluation of a person with back pain. Here are some of the tests that many doctors consider mandatory.

Straight Leg Lift Test. This is performed with a patient lying flat on the back with feet fully extended. The examiner lifts one leg at a time to see if there is any patient pain. If there is a sciatica problem, usually pain will shoot down the

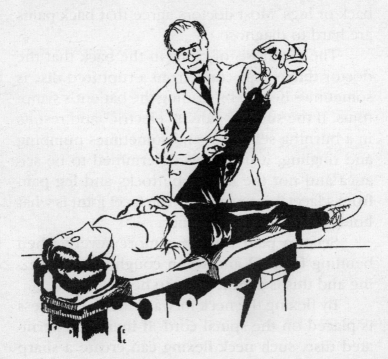

affected leg when it is lifted from about twenty-five to seventy-five degrees. When the leg is lifted this way it actually stretches the nerve roots at the spinal cord and they are put under increased tension which causes the pain. Both legs are lifted this way, one at a time.

Related Pain Test. If pain courses down one leg when the other leg is being raised, it is another indication of sciatica with the added problem of a disc fragment. In this case a piece of the herniated disc may have broken off and is pressing against the sciatic nerve root.

The Lasegue Test. Here the patient's ankle and foot are pushed up toward the knee. This will put further stress on the nerve roots and if there is a problem with a disc, will cause intense pain.

Neurological Examination of Leg. For this exam a pinwheel or other neurological tool is used to test any nerve problem in the leg, thigh or foot. Here too, reflexes at the back of the ankle and the knee will be tested and evaluated.

Motor Strength Test. The motor strength will be tested in the leg, ankle and foot in one or both legs and the results evaluated.

Lumbar Area Motion and Range Test. The range and motion of the lumbar spine area will be tested as well as the route of the sciatic nerve going down the leg for tenderness or spasming.

These tests will not only confirm or rule out a sciatic problem, but will help the examiner to figure out just which disc is affected.

OTHER TESTS

If none of the above methods show that there could be a herniated disc, the doctor has other tools.

The X-Ray. Taking X-rays of the lumbar region of your spine is a quick and inexpensive way to check for problems with your lower back; however, they simply can't detect a ruptured disc. That's because the regular X-ray shows bones, and bone structure; they can't show the soft tissue of which the disc is made.

What X-rays can show are other problems with your back and spine such as cancer, fractures in your spine or arthritis damage to the vertebrae. If your pain continues, your doctor may start the testing with an X-ray just to rule out other problems.

CAT Scan. The next test your doctor may try could be a computerized tomographic scan, CT or often called a CAT scan. Again it will pinpoint the lower back and the lumbar vertebrae since this is where sciatica pain is caused.

Most specialists say that a CAT scan can find

24

75% of herniated discs when they are taken properly. The CAT scan is not without some distortion and some disc problems may seem to be there when there is nothing wrong. But it's the best test we have right now.

How does it work?

A CAT scan is done in the radiology department of a hospital or clinic. It's an outpatient procedure and no hospitalization is required. The patient wears a hospital gown and is placed on a platform which is slowly moved into a large circular device that encloses the person. The CAT scan is painless.

As the patient is slowly drawn through the large tube, a scanner is taking millions of readings by special types of rays that result in a print out of a perfect picture of the area, in this case the spine. A computer prints out pictures of the area and a diagnosis is made.

The pictures from this machine will show the discs between the vertebrae and in about 75 percent of the cases the radiologist can determine if there is a herniated disc or not.

The scanner gives out cross sections of the spine less than a quarter of an inch thick. With the computer scanner the interior of the bones can be evaluated. The computer reconstructs the views of the scanner and comes up with the precise areas that the radiologists asks it to.

Yes, the CAT scan involves radiation, and since a session might take a half hour or more, some patients wonder about being over exposed to the radiation. Actually the radiation comes in brief strobes and an entire CAT scan will give a patient no more radiation exposure than four or five regular X-rays.

Magnetic Resonance Imaging. The MRI uses a magnetic field and radio waves to produce signals that are then converted into images of your body by a computer. The MRI is another method of testing for a herniated disc. Some specialists say the MRI is better at finding ruptured discs than the CAT scan. One drawback is the cost. An MRI can cost from about $600 to as much as $4,000 depending on what is tested and how long it takes.

Most MRI's will find a herniated disc in 90 percent of the cases.

The MRI is painless and there is no radiation exposure to worry about. It works through the use of magnetic rays which are harmless. Again, this is an outpatient procedure and no hospitalization is needed. There are no injections or medications and any risk factor is extremely low.

The MRI can show up cancer, infection and fractures in the spine as well as herniated discs.

Sometimes it can give a false image of a ruptured disc when it isn't there. The MRI and the CAT scan are the best diagnostic tools we have so far for the disc problem. Its use can mean no myelogram is needed.

The Myelogram. A myelogram is a test that uses a radiopague fluid that is injected directly into the spine cavities near a suspected ruptured disc or other spinal problems. The fluid is impervious to X-rays. Now the X-rays will show up many problems with the discs that a straight X-ray could not.

The myelogram can leave a patient with a headache and dizziness but some patients have no side effects. As with any invasive procedure, the myelogram carries with it a small element of risk to the patient. It is also uncomfortable for the patient.

Many doctors now would rather use a CAT scan than a myelogram because it is simpler, less invasive, easier on the patient and usually just as good or better results can be obtained.

MENSTRUAL SCIATIC PAIN

On some rare instances other causes can trigger sciatica pain. A case in point. A woman in Tokyo went to her doctor about sciatica pains coinciding with her menstrual cycle. She said she had severe right-side sciatica that began a day before her menstruation began, peaked two days into the cycle and then gradually ebbed away over the next fourteen days. After that she was pain free until two days before the next cycle.

The doctor's X-rays showed nothing. Her blood cell count, blood chemistry and erythrocyte sedimentation rate were all normal.

A CT scan of her lumbar spine showed a small disc herniation between the L5 and S1 vertebral levels. The doctor discounted this as the source of the pain.

Further CT scanning showed a large mass in the pelvic cavity. More testing showed it to be an endometrioma. The doctor shrank the endometrial cyst and the woman's sciatic symptoms vanished.

This cause of sciatica pain is rare, but if all else fails it could be an area to investigate.

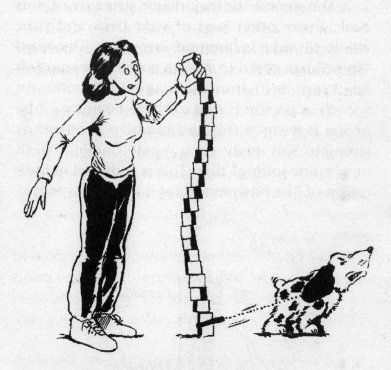

CHAPTER TWO:
WHAT IS YOUR SPINE?

Before we get into too much detail here about the sciatica problem and ways to handle it, let's do some basic training and take a good look at the spine—that's where this problem centers and we need to know as much about it as we can.

The spine is the major bone structure of your back. Every other part of your back and your whole rib cage is hung on this spine. The word "spine" has come to have a special meaning. It has crept into literature and into common speech. A person is said to "have no spine" if he or she is wishy washy and has no will power or strength. You might get a "spine tingling" thrill or a "spine jolting" ride. This is some small indication of just how important this spine is to us.

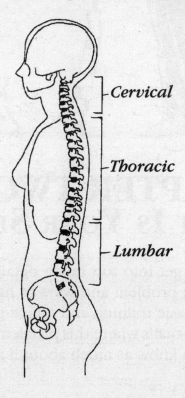

Cervical

Thoracic

Lumbar

THE VERTEBRAE

The back has one basic building block, it's called the vertebra.

It's a relatively small bone, only a few inches wide. However, this group of twenty-three vertebrae do a tremendous job of permitting the human body to bend and twist and do all sorts of complicated maneuvers without breaking. The word itself comes from the Latin word *vertere*, which means to turn.

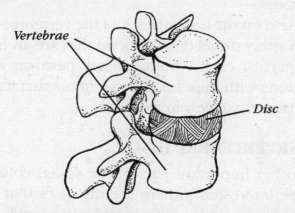

The vertebrae have been honed and sculptured and tailor made to their tasks down through millions of years of evolution into three dimensional building blocks that do at least four vital functions in your back.

Just like building blocks, the vertebrae are stacked up in order, some larger than others and each group designed for specific purposes. The stack of vertebrae form a strong column that is designed to support the considerable weight of the upper body.

The body of the vertebra is nearly circular in shape. It has a hole through it on the backside and these holes are all aligned to form a smooth vertical hole or tunnel from top to bottom. This is called the spinal canal and it contains and protects the spinal cord through which all of the major nerves from the brain run to the rest of the body.

Also on the back of each of the vertebrae are seven spiny projections of bone that are an integral part of each vertebra. They perform vital functions with muscles and ligaments that we're not concerned with in this study.

INTERVERTEBRAL DISCS

The other important part of the spinal column we are interested in here are the discs that are situated between the bottom and tops of each vertebra and cushion and serve as shock absorbers for the spine.

These "pillows" between the vertebrae are about a quarter of an inch in thickness, maybe more in some people and less in others, and they will also vary in width from one vertebra to the next depending where it is in the spinal column and how much pressure is on it.

These discs are what compress and expand to allow the spinal column to bend and shift with the stretching and work loads the muscles attached to it accept.

The discs will shrink in their thickness during the day when the body is pushing down on them for hours at a time. But at night they will be unpressured and will revert back to their original size. Some people are from a half to three quarters of an inch shorter after an active day, than they were when they got out of bed that morning.

Discs are composed not of bone but of a substance similar to the cartilage that forms your ears and nose. In the discs it is slightly yellowish and is called fibrocartilage.

The disc has two main parts, the inner core, a pulpy and soft mass named the *nucleus pulposus.* The outer part of the disc is made up of parallel fibers that are harder and hold the core in place. This is called the *annulus fibrosus.* Think of a jelly donut with the jelly the core and the outside of the donut holding the jelly in as the outer ring.

A car tire is another example of the disc. Just as a tire has pressure inside, so does the core of the disc. The discs are more than eighty percent water. This is what permits them to hold the pressure and to be elastic so they can let the spine bend on call. The disc can change shape rather drastically and then when the pressure is removed by the spine, the disc returns to its original shape.

The high water content lets the disc absorb blows and jolts to the upper body. That's the reason the discs are called the shock absorbers for the spine.

THE RIGHT CONNECTION

The vertebrae are joined together in this vertical stack by the facet joints. These fairly flat surfaces slide over each other to some extent to permit some movement. By the same factor, they also limit how far you can bend or twist your back.

All of your vertebrae are joined together in three places: the main disc joint and the two auxiliary facet joints at the rear. Any of these joints can cause a lot of back trouble.

ALL IN A STACK

The vertebrae all stacked up in the right order are called the human backbone. Medical people divide this stack into three main sections. The top six vertebrae are called the cervical ones. These serve the neck and end about at the top of the shoulders.

The next twelve are named the thoracic vertebrae. These go from the shoulders almost to the bottom of the rib cage. The other five bones and discs are named the lumbar vertebrae and extend to just above the hip bones.

The lumbar vertebrae are the ones that we are the most concerned with, since this is where the majority of the problems occur that result in sciatica.

If you looked at a spinal column from the front, it would appear to be a straight vertical stack of bones with no curves to the right or left. However if you look at the same spine from the side, you'll see that it does have several curves.

Through the neck area there is the cervical curve which swings slightly backwards from the chest. Just below that in the thoracic vertebrae the curve reverses itself and now swings outward toward the chest. Just below the rib cage the lumbar curve swings the spine again toward the back. Below the hip bones the sacral curve moves the spine all the way to the tail bone in a forward curve again. These curves must be in the right places and in the right form for your spine to function normally.

THE SPINAL NERVES

We are vitally concerned with the nerves that run through this vertical spinal canal. Those nerves are what send many men and women straight up the wall with sciatica pain.

This canal runs the entire length of the spinal column from the base of the brain downward. Inside this sheath in the canal run a sensitive bundle of hundreds of nerve cells and fibers. They form a group about as thick as a man's small finger. This group of nerves is the super highway of communications from the brain to the body.

Nerves branch off from the main stem to meet the needs of every body part. They go at regular intervals in pairs on each side of each of the vertebrae. They are called nerve roots. There are thirty-one pairs of nerve roots emanating from the spinal cord.

Each set of nerves is designed to service a specific part of the body. They soon branch out and combine and branch again until that part of the body is completely serviced with nerve endings. For example the nerves between the fourth and fifth neck vertebrae serve the muscles that

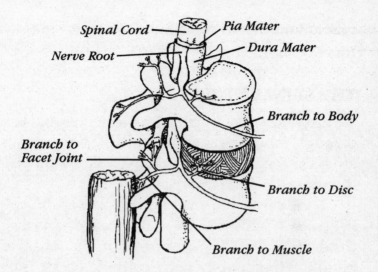

Spinal Cord — Pia Mater — Dura Mater — Nerve Root — Branch to Body — Branch to Facet Joint — Branch to Disc — Branch to Muscle

let you move your shoulders and upper arms.

The nerves exiting from between the fourth and fifth lumbar vertebrae leave the hips and go down each leg to activate the hips and knees. Those from between the fifth lumbar and the sacrum let us move our feet.

These nerves that control the legs and feet combine high up and bundle together as they work down from the hips are called the sciatic nerve. This nerve is where the trouble can come from if you suffer from sciatica pain.

So, that's the human spine, a marvelously wonderful structure that we're going to be talking about a lot during this study of sciatic pain and what you can do about it.

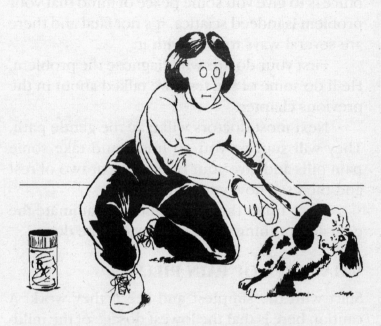

CHAPTER THREE:
TREATING SCIATICA THE TRADITIONAL WAY

When truly painful sciatica hits, the first thing you think of is to go to a doctor to be sure what you have. Sometimes serious pain in almost any part of the body can mean cancer or some other dangerously serious ailment. You want to rule out those causes at once. This first stop at a doctor's office is to give you some peace of mind that your problem is indeed sciatica, it's not fatal and there are several ways to deal with it.

First your doctor will diagnose the problem. He'll do some of the tests we talked about in the previous chapter.

Next most doctors will take the gentle path. They will suggest you go home and take some pain pills and give your back a day or two of rest and then see how you feel.

Many times this will reduce or eliminate the pain and nothing more will need to be done.

WHAT TYPE OF PAIN PILLS?

Start with the simplest and see if they work. A caution here is that the lowest dosage of the mildest pill you can take that does the job is the one to stick with. None of these pain pills should be taken without a doctor's advice for more than ten days.

The simplest is any of the common aspirins on the market. From the supermarket bottle of 500 to the fancy wrapped package of a name brand, all do about the same thing. They are anti-inflammatory analgesics that help make tissue repair as well as work on your pain.

Others in this class include the buffered aspirin, Anacin and Excedrin. This group include the newer ibuprofen tablets on the market such as Advil and Motrin and the naproxen sodium tablets such as Aleve. All of them will help reduce pain and at the same time help start the repair procedures in the body to patch up your ruptured disc or inflammation around the disc.

These are all non-prescription medications. Be sure to follow the directions on the box for dosage and length of use. The main advantage of these drugs is that they contain no opiates, they are not addictive and this is highly important to those with chronic back pain.

MUSCLE RELAXANTS

When you start talking about medications to relax the muscles including those in your back that are torturing you, you get into the realm of prescription drugs that do contain narcotics. The big danger here is getting addicted to the pills so you can't do without them.

These include drugs such as Percodan and Rbaxisal and Tylenol-2, Tylenol-3 and Tylenol-4. Tylenol-2 contains fifteen mg of codeine. The 3 Tylenol has thirty mg of codeine and the 4 has sixty mg of codeine. Codeine is one of the drugs that is easy to become addicted to.

A note of warning. If you use more than one

doctor, such as a GP and a neurologist, be sure that you tell each what medications you are taking so they are not duplicated and so no medications are prescribed that will cause great pain and suffering when taken at the same time. Anytime you get a new prescription filled, tell your pharmacist what other medications you're taking and ask him if any of them should not be taken at the same time. He'll know.

The rule with any medication: use as little as you can to get the job done, and use it for as short a time as possible.

CHRONIC OPIOID THERAPY

While we're talking about drugs and medications, there's a term you need to know: Chronic Opioid. What this means is the practice of prescribing intensely dangerous drugs such as morphine and high potency codeine and any of a dozen other effective but highly addictive drugs to a patient with back pain. This is sometimes done by doctors who can figure out no other way to stop the patient's pain.

Doctors who use this therapy say they are extremely careful to choose the patient carefully for chronic opioid. They say there is a certain percentage of back pain patients who can undergo this therapy with no substance abuse and no addiction.

That must be a small percentage. Even if the patient doesn't develop an addiction there is still the problem of severe side effects. They include persistent constipation, insomnia, lowered sexual desire and function and even trouble thinking clearly and focusing on current time.

Here is one doctor's check list he uses before prescribing any chronic opioid treatment:

◆ It should be used only after all other reasonable attempts at pain control have not worked.
◆ If the patient has any history of drug abuse, this therapy can't be used.
◆ One prescribing doctor must take personal responsibility for the patient and follow up on him or her weekly.
◆ Any patient must give an informed consent prior to starting this treatment. Make it a written consent form.
◆ Dosages should be used on an around-the-clock basis.
◆ If the patient does not receive partial pain relief after the first few low doses, this treatment should be stopped.
◆ Any evidence of drug abuse or addiction should be recognized in the patient and the treatments stopped.

BED REST

Most older books and manuals on back problems tout bed rest for from two weeks up to a month as a basic treatment for many patients. Now doctors have changed that policy. Specialists currently say that one or perhaps two days of bed rest after a shattering bout with sciatica or other back problems is as much as you should do.

Bed rest doesn't mean total immobility. Rest your back, but don't worry about getting out of bed two or three times a day. Going to the bathroom is fine but get right back to bed for that day or two.

Bed rest is good for many of the backache problems beside sciatica. But too much bed rest can cause problems. Some regimens just ten or fifteen years ago called for six to eight weeks of bed rest. Most doctors now say that this is far too much; one to three days is more realistic.

Too much time in bed can cause all sorts of problems including weakening of the muscles and a tendency to soften the bones. It can cause depression, stomach and bowel upsets, loss of bone and mineral tissue, blood clots in the legs, weakening of the spine's discs, cartilage and ligaments.

Get up for meals during these bed resting times, but don't over do it. Remember that you can over protect your back and it can lead to problems down the line.

THE PHYSIOTHERAPIST ENTERS THE SCENE

After your doctor has checked you, done tests to be sure there are no serious causes of your back pain such as a tumor or a cancer, and determines that there is no need for surgery, most medical doctors then pass the patient on to a physical therapist. These physiotherapists are schooled in a variety of methods and treatments to help you get rid of your back pain. These vary as widely as the therapists and range all over the scale. Here are some of them and how they might be used to reduce or eliminate your own back problems.

CAN CORSETS, BRACES AND TRACTION HELP?

Opinion is divided in the medical world over these three types of treatment for many back problems including sciatica. Since the back was not functioning the way it should, which probably led to the back problem in the first place, why not use a corset or a brace to keep it in the right position?

An old-fashioned woman's corset could do

the trick, but these are harder to find these days than an honest politician. Even the use of one for a long period of time as a stand in for firm abdominal muscles can have detrimental effects. Some say that such a corset will tend to take over the functions of these muscles and can let the muscles weaken and shrink away.

Braces

The same problem can come with braces, however the braces are designed to support certain areas and are less restrictive, so they will adversely affect fewer of these vital muscles.

What braces? These are called lumbar or lumbosacral braces. They go from the pelvis to the middle of the rib cage and come with a variety of elements running down and across the body. Some of the braces extend down to the side of the hip. With such a brace on, the person wearing it is constantly reminded to restrict his sudden movements.

If you or your medical advisor decides that a brace will help you, there are two that could do the job. One is the Boston Brace and the other the Raney Flexion Jacket.

These braces are designed for good abdominal compression and for a minor flexed lumbar spine. This lumbar flexing can decrease the backward bulge of a disc and relive some of the pressure on the lumbar spine's rear elements.

Any lumbar brace you buy is going to be expensive. Just the nature of the beasts. These are not used as much today as they were in the past and you might have trouble finding them in some areas. Be sure this is what you need before you go this route.

They have some other drawbacks. Braces can irritate bony pominences in your back as well as your skin. Sometimes a back brace will cause more pain instead of lessening it.

Traction

Traction is usually used in a hospital situation where ropes pull one part of your body one way while other ropes pull it the opposite direction. Once used extensively for sciatica, but after several clinical studies on traction, it was determined that it does little if any good at all for sciatica and most back problems. It just doesn't do any good.

TENS

This acronym stands for Transcutaneous Electrical Nerve Stimulation. Back in the 1960's with the advent of electrodes, the use of electricity to reduce pain had a surge of popularity. Then electrodes were surgically put into painful areas of the back and activated with low charges of electricity.

That quickly led to the creation of a TENS machine. This is now a portable battery powered machine that can be worn around the waist that has electrodes that are taped to the skin on the back in the pain area. The electric current is delivered from the battery pack on an on-demand need by the patient.

TENS machines are of two types. In one the current resembles a buzz, the other is more like a gentle and nudging electric shock. The electrodes are placed on the back in a number of places until the best spots are located. Then they are left in that productive area.

Often used for chronic back pain, the TENS treatment is said to give relief from pain in about a third of the patients. Experts say that the electric current's high frequency stimulates the large sensory fibers. This lessens the patient feeling the pain as it travels along the smaller sensory fibers.

TRIGGER POINT INJECTIONS

Sometimes pain in the back can be pin pointed by the patient. By pressing on this area it triggers more pain. These are called trigger points and can cause pains in other areas far from the back.

Some therapists believe that injections of

local anesthetic such as cortisone or saline can relieve the pain. This often will give quick relief but it is not permanent. During such relief, you may be able to use other methods of treatment that were not practical before such as applying moist heat or doing exercises.

There is no solid evidence that such injections will work for everyone, however if it works for you, be thankful. Be sure the needles are sterile and the injections are given correctly.

ULTRASOUND

Your physical therapist or doctor may suggest ultrasound in some situations to reduce pain and help healing. Ultrasound delivers high frequency sound waves of over a million cycles per second into targeted tissue. This is the same as ultrasound used for diagnostic work, but the wattage is much lower and the heat generated is less.

The ultrasound vibrates individual cells in the body. This is thought to cut down on the pain by activating the large sensory fibers so the relatively few pain messages working along the small fibers are not as recognized—hence less felt pain.

Ultrasound can also help break down scar tissue and at the same time activate new connective tissue. Ultrasound will also change the characteristic of the cell walls. With heightened per-

49

meability, the cell can rid itself of waste products easier and nutrients can be absorbed quicker. This means an inflamed area will see healing take place faster.

HOT AND COLD PACKS

Hot packs, moist or dry, should not be used on a new injury, and that applies to a hurt back or a sciatic screamer. But after the injury is moderated, hot packs will help bring new blood into the region and help healing. The heat is soothing to any injury and with the increase in blood supply and oxygen, it will help decrease muscle tension. Heat can also stimulate the large sensory fibers and decrease the perception of pain.

Cold packs are often used to reduce swelling. There is little swelling in a sciatic pain situation, but the cold pack can still be helpful. It reduces the circulation to the area when used. If it is alternated with a hot pack the new infusion of blood will be greater than with the hot pack alone. If you find a hot pack is more painful than soothing, try switching to a cold pack. One man said he used a cold pack because he couldn't feel a thing when he had his back frozen stiff from an ice pack. Generally an ice pack should not be placed directly on the skin and should not be used for more than fifteen minutes at a time.

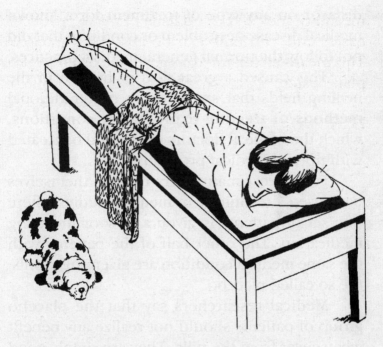

CHAPTER FOUR:
TREATING SCIATICA WITH NON-TRADITIONAL METHODS

A GENERAL POSITIONING

For a great many years in this country and abroad, the medical community has looked with extreme disfavor on any type of treatment for a known medical disease or problem or condition that did not follow the normal general medical practices.

This caused a great deal of friction in the healing fields that specialize in non-traditional methods of treating many bodily conditions, which the medical doctors say should be treated with normal medical procedures.

For a great many years doctors themselves have used a technique in medical studies where one set of patients is given a new or in-testing medication. The other half of the patients with the same medical condition are given sugar pills, the so called placebo.

Medical researchers say that the placebo group of patients should not realize any benefit whatsoever from the pills. They are simply good tasting sugar pills. Much to the surprise and sometimes chagrin of researchers, there always is a percentage of the placebo patients who show improvement when taking the inert sugar pills in a closely controlled, double blind, testing situation.

It has come to be known as the placebo effect, and is pushed into the realm of the psychiatrist who tells us that some people can effect "cures" and "benefits" and "improvements" in their condition in a great variety of ailments, simply by believing that they are receiving medication that will generate these improvements in their condition.

Closely allied with the placebo effect is the psychosomatic situation. Psychosomatic is simply the result of bodily symptoms that are caused by mental or emotional disturbances. You've heard of a psychosomatic illness — when a person starts to believe that he or she has a physical problem and they absolutely *know they have it* and soon they develop the physical symptoms of that disease or problem. Medical doctors can become extremely mixed up by such symptoms only to find with tests that the person actually doesn't have the disease at all.

You may have heard of a false pregnancy, where a woman wants to have a child with such great emotional desire, that she actually misses her periods and her belly starts to swell and her breasts enlarge — but there is no pregnancy. This is a psychosomatic condition.

What this is saying is that in many ways the mind can have a physical effect on the body. Medical experts have long believed this. People can "think themselves sick". The whole problem area of stress is a problem of the mind affecting the body. This area of mind and body relationships is not an exact science and by this time, many traditional medical men take this attitude: "If it works, if it helps heal the body and is beneficial to the patient, let it happen."

This whole subject of alternative medicine, or non-traditional treatment of conditions and even diseases, carries with it this codicil:

"If it works, use it. If a non-traditional treatment helps the patient to get better, even if it's only psychologically, it's a benefit to the patient."

A man once said that if a person is simply lazy, a psychologist can probably cure him and get him back to work. But if that same man isn't working because he has a broken leg, he better go see a medical doctor to get the broken bone set.

Put this down as a type of disclaimer. There are millions of people who believe passionately in non-traditional forms of healing of mind and body. If you aren't one of them, look at these "different" forms of healing and maintaining your spine and your back with a good deal of common sense. Some of them might work for you. Some of them might trigger a placebo effect that will be tremendously worth while for you. Some of them may have inherent curative powers. Some of them might not work at all for you.

You must be the final judge and jury. It all boils down to this. If it's traditional or some far out methodology, if it works for you, run with it and don't do a lot of worrying about why.

MASSAGE

There is no clinical proof through studies by recognized experts that massage can do any good whatsoever for sciatica or back pain. On the other hand there are hundreds of thousands of men and women who swear by a good massage as a way to gain relief, even if temporary, from any number of back pains and aches and troubles including sciatica.

In this enlightened age, no type of remedy, no matter how unusual or strange, can be denounced or ridiculed if it works for some people. If it works, it's a factor. Massage works for many people in a number of different ways.

One expert masseuse says that massage helps contracted muscles relax. That means the relaxed muscles let blood circulation increase. The greater circulation gets rid of toxic wastes faster including lactic acid from body tissues. Muscles that are contracted produce lactic acid, and a build up of lactic acid can produce pain.

How else might massage help with back pain? An injury in the back can mean that some muscles go into spasm to protect the injured area. The spasm becomes a kind of splint giving that protection. Once the injured area is healed, the "splint" of spasming muscle should relax. Often this doesn't happen.

Massage can be used to help relax the muscle. However since the spasm was in place for some time, it can often return with the slightest increase in pressure or stress on the former injury. A number of massages may be needed to permanently relax that particular muscle and keep it in a natural state.

Some of the best massage therapists gladly work with, not against, medical doctors. Many will encourage their patients with back problems to exercise and improve their posture.

If it works for you, use massage.

There is a growing belief in the healing world that simply being touched by another person can have nourishing and healing benefits. The idea of touching as a method for pain relief is becoming more recognized. One massage therapist said: "An exchange of energy is involved in the touching aspect of massage. It can help a person feel less alone and more connected to the world."

What about Chinese Massage? The Chinese type of massage has been used for over 2,000 years to cure disease in China. Massage for pain relief is one type of Chinese massage. This natural and physical type therapy works on channels, acupoints, pain-relief points and affected parts of the body with various manipulations to relieve symptoms of pain and to cure some diseases.

This method follows the traditional rules of Chinese medicine which is "to cure disease, you must cure its root."

Chinese medicine deals with Ying and Yang and with the two essential substances, Qu and blood.

Two examples of how this all works. However, if you want to get into Chinese massage, you should find a whole book on the subject and study it carefully. It's an entirely different world from the Western way of thinking.

Now an example: What about sciatica or chronic back pain? Chinese Massage says that back pain comes from an injury or an invasion of Cold and Damp. It could also be the result of weakness of the kidneys, neurosis, exhaustion or frequent sexual intercourse.

The purpose of this treatment is to strengthen the back and the kidneys. It also improves Qu-blood flow and expels Cold and Damp.

What should you do for this problem?

Working with acupoints on each side of the back of the neck, you should squeeze them with thumb and fore finger. Do this ten times. Then locate the acupoints on the back of each shoulder half way between the neck and the outside of the shoulder. Squeeze each of these points for twenty to thirty times.

Step two here is to open channels in the back region. These acupoints are near the bottom of the back and low down and on one side. Squeeze these points in sequence forty to fifty times.

The Chinese Massage for the back covers nine points such as the two above with definite areas of the body to squeeze and massage.

If this type of therapy interests you, by all means get a good book on Chinese Massage and start learning how to do it.

THE RELAXATION RESPONSE TECHNIQUE

There may be a way you can reduce the pain of your sciatica or your back simply by doing nothing. Well, almost nothing. Try relaxation.

Get in a comfortable sitting position. Maintain your breathing in a normal way. Close your eyes and repeat a favorite word or phrase, perhaps simply "one" or "relaxing". Repeat this word over and over again pushing all other thoughts and stimuli out of your mind.

Concentrate on this one word and clear your mind of all else for five minutes, saying your key word over and over again in your mind. Try hard not to go to sleep during this exercise.

Dr. Herb Benson of Boston calls this procedure "the relaxation response."

This technique is similar to many of the world's religious prayer rituals, and is almost identical to the transcendental meditation with the exception that the one key word replaces the mantra or the prayer.

Will it work for you? Nobody claims to know all the benefits of this type of relaxation response, but most experts agree that it can reduce stress and in many cases reduce the severity of pain. Some think that such a regimen helps the brain and the spinal cord to release endorphins, that are known to help relax and bring about a state of well being. Endorphins are natural pain killers and thought to be the body's naturally produced version of morphine.

BIOFEEDBACK

This method of pain relief is not as popular as it was only a few years ago. Some people and practitioners still swear by it. It is a system of using an electronic sensor to pick up the electrical responses from a muscle that contracts in association with tension. The tension in your muscles, the temperature of your fingers and the amount of sweat you produce can all be used to show muscle tension. The person using it learns to relax and to relax the muscle as a voluntary and controlled response to the feedback. When this works, the relaxed muscle will reduce the pain.

HYDROTHERAPY

Some doctors and homeopaths advise the use of hydrotherapy as a means of reducing the inflammation associated with sciatica and in many cases reducing the pain. Water is available to everyone and can be used effectively to help reduce back pain. Most people think of exercising in a heated pool as a hydrotherapy method. This is a good one, however any use of water is hydrotherapy.

If you have hot and cold running water in your home, you can use this special hydrotherapy technique. It's called hot and cold formentations by some and it is used this way.

Take two towels, large enough to be folded to three thicknesses and cover the affected area you want to treat, in this case your lower back. Soak one towel in hot tap water and wring it out, fold into three thicknesses and apply to your back or have someone else put on the towel while you're lying on your stomach.

Leave this towel in place for three minutes. During that time take the second towel and soak it in cold tap water or ice water. Wring it out. Replace the hot towel after three minutes with the cold one for a minute. Now soak the hot towel again and repeat the rotation of hot and cold. This procedure can be done for twenty to thirty minutes to help relieve the pain and promote healing.

How does it work? The hot towel heats up and expands all of the capillaries in the affected area, which at once draws more blood than usual into the heated area. The blood helps to repair any damage to the spinal area and fight inflammation. Then the cold towel comes and drives the blood away. A minute later the hot towel comes and fresh blood surges into the area.

This infusion of new blood every minute or so will help your back to heal and to reduce the pain.

Other forms of hydrotherapy include hot/cold showers, and a warm bath. Don't let the bath be too hot or it will reduce the effect. You can also use Epsom salts in a warm bath or various herbs for a herbal bath.

ACUPUNCTURE

Acupuncture is said to have been practiced in China for over 5,000 years. It came to the United States in the 1970's with a bang and held a lot of popular appeal, but then it faded and almost died out. Now it has been Westernized and many medical doctors use it in their regular practice.

Just what is acupuncture?

Acupuncture is the placement of needles into what are called acupuncture points where the Chinese say the blood and bodily energy converge. Western doctors who studied this new technique quickly discovered that the 800 Chinese points correspond roughly with the western physicians understanding of the neural structures. This meant that Western doctors could use their understanding of the neural points as the basis for acupuncture treatments. They did not have to study the Chinese system and learn a whole new set of 800 points on the human body. Now a Western physician could utilize acupuncture as part of a treatment using Western medical principles and choosing the points for the needles on an anatomical basis.

Needles. The very idea gives some people the shakes and run-for-the-woods impulses. The needles used in acupuncture are much thinner than those used these days for shots. They are thinner since they don't have to be hollow.

They also are rounded on the end. This makes them less painful than an injection needle. An injection needle point must be a puncture type that will slash through tissue. Also remember with a shot, much of the pain comes not from the needle, but from the solution being injected into your body. If you get a shot of penicillin it will really hurt. If you get a tetanus shot it will hurt and you'll be able to taste the serum almost immediately. Needles for acupuncture come in various lengths for different uses.

The traditional method of using needles is to insert them at the proper place and then twirl them. Now a device is used that will twirl the needles and at the same time it will electrically stimulate the area with different levels of electrical current and intensity. This is called electroacupuncture and does not hurt, rather it gives the patient a pulsating feeling.

There are two theories about how acupuncture works. The older one is that the needles stimulate the large nerve fibers which send sensations such as temperature and touch to the brain. The smaller nerve fibers send the pain signals to the brain.

The theory is that the large fibers are overstimulated until they overload. Somehow this overload acts as a valve that also shuts down the small nerve fibers in the area. If the nerve can't send the pain signal to the brain, the patient doesn't feel the pain.

The other theory is that the human brain can produce powerful pain killers called endorphins and enkephalins. Some experts say that the use of acupuncture will stimulate the brain to produce these two natural opiate pain killers.

The idea is that the acupuncture stimulates one specific area, the brain gets the message and quickly sends endorphins by way of the nervous system back to the spot where the acupuncture was given. This then turns off the pain and the patient feels better.

Does it work?

That you'll have to figure out for yourself through trial and error. If nothing else seems to satisfy your pain reduction needs, give acupuncture a try. It can't hurt anything.

Will it work on sciatica?

One patient had serious sciatica pain and could find no relief. She went to an acupuncturist who was also a medical doctor. He used ten different sized needles from one to three inches long. Two were inserted on each side of the spine near the point where the L5 vertebra nerve roots come out of the spinal canal. Two more went in at the S2 area with one on each side of the spine.

The other six needles were positioned down the left leg of the woman where she felt the intense sciatica pain. The needles were stimulated with electrical current.

After the first thirty minute treatment she felt better. After four treatments a week apart, the sciatica pain was almost gone.

Acupuncture is not a mysterious end-all for pain. It may not completely stop a pain, but many medicines don't completely stop pain either.

Some states have strict laws regarding acupuncture, other states are more lenient. You may wish to check the legal ramifications in your area before contacting an acupuncturist. One rule of thumb: if there are ads for acupuncturists in your local telephone yellow pages, they are probably legal and licensed in your area.

ACUPRESSURE AND SCIATICA

Acupressure is the fraternal twin to acupuncture. Basically the only difference is that acupressure uses finger and hand pressure on the pressure points of the body instead of the needles of acupuncture.

What pressure?

Thumb pressure is done with the ball of the thumb. The thrust is perpendicular to the pressure point. It can be a back and forth method or a circular motion with the side of the thumb and nail.

Other techniques include the use of finger

pressure, grasping skin between finger and thumb, tapping a pressure point with fist, knuckle, palm or finger, rubbing, clenched fist rocking and the pinching of flesh.

How does acupressure work on the body?

Acupressure breaks the reflex arc between the pressure points just beneath the skin and those various organs to which it communicates. It rearranges the forces of the body that channel pain and hurt in a part of the body. This tends to sedate the automatic nervous system which was complaining, and a more normal state is achieved.

Acupressure increases the flow of arterial blood.

Acupressure stimulates the endocrine gland.

Acupressure stimulates lymph gland and venous drainage.

Acupressure releases waste products from musculature.

Acupressure helps to produce physiological peace and mental relaxation.

Acupressure lowers the pain and the hurting.

This isn't intended to be a course in acupressure. Whole books are written on it. For example there are over 200 pressure points on the body you'll need to know about, eight on the face alone.

How does acupressure apply to sciatica and other back pain?

For sciatica, acupressure regimens call for searching for hypersensitive points in these locations:

◆ middle of the thigh.
◆ in the sciatic notch of the pelvic bones.
◆ at the fifth lumbar vertebra.
◆ the crest of the ileum in back.

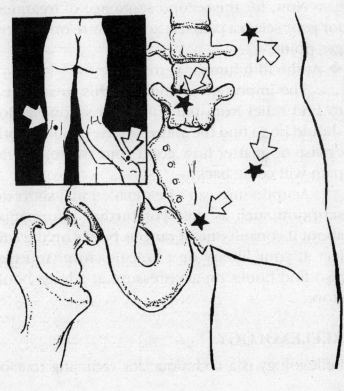

◆ at the outside of the ankle bones.

◆ in the popliteal space behind the knee.

Now, to treat for sciatica pain in the lower back, the buttocks and the legs and ankles, apply finger or thumb pressure at these points:

◆ At the crest of the ileum on your back.

◆ In the sciatic notch in the pelvic bones.

◆ In the middle of the thigh.

◆ In the popliteal space behind the knee.

◆ At the outside ankle bones.

Now, for the second sequence of treatment for your sciatica pain use acupressure on this trigger point:

◆ At the fifth lumbar vertebra.

The important element in this treatment is to find relief from the pain. The second action should be to find the source of the problem, otherwise no matter how good your treatment, the pain will come back.

Acupressure can't be detailed in a short description such as this. For further information about it consult one of various books on the subject at your library or a holistic store. You may also find books on acupressure at a large bookstore.

REFLEXOLOGY

Reflexology is a technique for reducing tension

and promoting well being. It is entirely non-invasive and works on many of the same principles as acupuncture and acupressure. Reflexology deals with the use of hand pressure on specific parts of the hands and feet only. A reflexology chart of the reflex points in the foot is similar in many ways to a chart in an acupuncture manual showing the foot's pressure points.

Reflexology is said to be a completely safe form of therapy besides being a relaxing and pleasant experience.

Purpose:

The purpose of reflexology is to normalize the body's functioning, to help break down tension and stress. It also can improve nerve functioning and increase the blood supply all through the body.

How does it work?

Reflexology strives to correct three factors in the body: congestion, inflammation and tension. The reflexology experts say that congestion can lead to growths in the body, inflammation means such conditions as colitis and sinusitis. Tension can mean a lowering of the efficiency of the immune system.

To create these benefits, reflexology is intended to improve the body's circulation and to help it by speeding up the elimination of waste products and toxins. Reflexology is also said to stimulate the release of endorphins to help control the perception of pain.

Proponents say that reflexology works the best when it is used for the whole body, not for a specific pain or problem. That way it improves the entire body's function which helps with the natural healing processes where they are needed.

What about Sciatica?

Experts on reflexology say this is the treatment for sciatica:

Begin by supporting the right foot with the right hand and use the index and third fingers of your left hand to work up the area just behind the ankle for about three inches. Repeat this pressure treatment three times. Then change feet and do the same thing on the left foot supporting it with the left hand and using the right hand for the application of pressure.

The procedure should continue with treatments for the hips and pelvis.

Do this by holding the right foot in an outward direction with your left hand. Use four fingers of your right hand to massage around the edge of the heel forward and then down. Repeat this pressure three times, then move to the other foot and repeat the process.

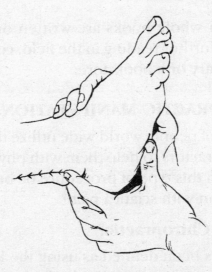

For hand reflexology for the spine do this:

For the reflex points for your spine on your right hand, work along the line from the base of your thumb, straight across the bottom of your hand, then up the length of your thumb. Do this three times for no more than seven seconds each. Repeat the pressure on your left hand.

For treatment for the spinal area on the foot:

Hold the top of the right foot with your left hand. Then use your right thumb to work up the reflex points along the right side of the bottom of the foot all the way to the big toe. Repeat three times, then do the other foot the same way.

Reflexology is not an exact science. What might help one person may not affect another at all. Again whole books are written on this subject. For further reading in the field, contact your local library or a bookstore.

CHIROPRACTIC MANIPULATION

Millions of people world wide utilize the services of chiropractors to help them with physical problems. Can this type of procedure be beneficial to the person with sciatica pain?

What is Chiropractic?

It has been defined as using the knowledge of the nerve functions of the body in conjunction with the laws of anatomy and physiology to help produce normal nerve functions through the development of a plan for application of this skill to the spinal column.

Many of the chiropractors of today are well educated persons with six years of study behind them including a year of internship in a chiropractic facility. Their specialty is the spine. Their basic tool of operation is the manipulation of the spine.

A chiropractor is not permitted to prescribe drugs or any prescription medications. He can't draw blood or do any invasive procedures. Chiropractors can order X-rays taken and evaluate them. They can also utilize ultrasound treatments.

For years there has been a conflict between the chiropractors and the medical doctors. The chiropractors say the doctors are drug pushers and slicers and cutters. The medical doctors say the chiropractors try to make differential diagnoses of the back and back pain without adequate training, examination skills, knowledge or experience.

What do the chiropractors say?

(From chiropractic literature for the patient)

"Your spinal adjustment treatment depends on the cause of your sciatica. During a spinal adjustment, your chiropractor gently presses on your spine to relieve irritated nerves and increase movement in your joints."

"The chiropractic approach to disc problems is to help restore better motion and position to the spinal joint. Besides reducing disc bulging, better spinal function helps reduce inflammation and begins the slow process of healing the surrounding soft tissues."

"The chiropractic approach is to use carefully directed and controlled pressure to remove the interference from spinal structures. These chiropractic "adjustments" can be quite effective in reducing nerve irritation and its associated pain.

"Sciatica, like other health problems that can be traced to the spine, often responds dramatically to the restoration of normal spinal function through chiropractic care."

"Spinal adjustment can reduce the pain and facilitate healing. If yours is a bulging or degenerated disc, you may lie on your side as your chiropractor pushes gently down on the lower back to relieve the pressure on pinched nerves. If yours is a herniated disc, you may lie on your stomach as your chiropractor gently applies traction downward at the waist to reduce further injury to the disc. After adjustment, ice may be recommended for the first forty-eight hours. Your chiropractor may also use deep heat or ultrasound to help alleviate inflammation and pain. A lumbar support may be prescribed for either a distorted or herniated disc."

Just What is Manipulation?

The therapeutic mainstay of those who call themselves chiropractors is manipulation. This has been described as "an assisted passive motion applied to the spinal facet joints and sacroiliac joints."

An expert put it his way. "There's a stiff joint and you manipulate it and that makes it move. This increases the range of motion. A mobile joint is less likely to be painful than a stiff joint."

Physically, just what happens during manipulation?

The key words to remember here are "Range Of Motion", or ROM. Near the end of a joint's normal physiological range of motion is a buffer zone. Next to that is an elastic shield. This fiber shield has a spring like feel which is created by a negative pressure inside the joint's capsule. This pressure helps stabilize a joint.

When the parts of a joint are pressured beyond this elastic shield by manipulation, they come apart with a cracking sound. This is manipulation. The cracking is caused by the sudden escape of gases inside the synovial fluid of the joint's capsule. Another word for it is cavitation. Such bubbles of gas can be seen on an X-ray right after manipulation. They are usually absorbed within 30 minutes.

For that time, the elastic shield between the buffer zone and the paraphysiological ROM is not there. This leaves more room in the joint space and that makes the joint unstable. No more manipulation of this joint is safe. After the gases are absorbed back into the joint, it becomes normal again.

That is what manipulation is.

Does Manipulation Work?

As in any profession, there are all shades and types of chiropractors. Some guarantee you the moon making great claims of success. Others are more conservative.

One chiropractor says he'd rather treat people with sudden back pain than those with chronic pain. He says he can adjust a patient's back who has chronic back pain and he'll feel great for twenty minutes, but then the patient is right back where he was.

On the other hand, with a person who has made a sudden wrong move and has a fixated or frozen joint, a chiropractor can really help. After the inflammation has gone down, such a joint many times remains frozen. This chiropractor says his treatments help unfreeze the joint and the patient is back to normal.

Some chiropractors imply that their manipulation may also affect diseases of internal organs. Is this justified? Most experts agree that manipulation can accelerate the body's blood flow and heart rate. However beyond that there is no evidence that supports the idea that manipulation can have any effect whatsoever on general health or any visceral pathology, diseases or conditions.

Another problem many people find with chiropractors is their programs that call for preventive manipulation of patients when they are pain free. The extended plans of patient care that include twelve and up to twenty-four visits for treatment of an out of alignment spine are also looked upon by many in the medical community as a money wasting over-treatment by fast talking chiropractors.

See A Medical Doctor, Too

One major concern of medical doctors is that when a patient is treated by a chiropractor the patient is getting only a partial diagnosis of any potential problems. Most chiropractors are not trained to make a diagnosis of all of the factors that might be producing a symptom.

Most doctors suggest that after you see your chiropractor, you also see your family doctor to check further for other complications from your back pain or other causes. There are several serious medical problems that can radiate pain into the back or down the arm that have nothing to do with either the back or the arm.

This is what worries medical doctors. They say such diseases that can be missed by chipractors looking at back pain include an expanding aortic aneurysm, angina, paget's disease, goiter or a thyroid problem.

Many of today's better trained chiropractors agree with the idea that they should work in conjunction with medical doctors to be sure that all of the problems can be investigated when a patient has back or sciatica pain.

So Will Manipulation Help Your Sciatica?

It might and it might not. Here are four ways that many experts say manipulation can affect your back pain:

◆ Manipulation can improve the mobility between two vertebrae which will reduce the temporary inflammation that happens as a result of a locked spinal joint.

◆ Manipulation can help the smaller spinal muscles attaching one vertebra to another to relax which can reduce spasming and the pain that accompanies it.

◆ Manipulation can reduce the nerve irritation as a result of the improved mobility of the vertebra.

◆ Manipulation can cause the body to increase the release of endorphins, the body's natural pain killer, which can help relieve the pain of sciatica.

When Not to Have Manipulation

Chiropractors typically do not do any manipulations if their examination or X-rays show that there is any evidence of bone fractures, infection, cancer, severe arthritis or other possible conditions that would be aggravated by manipulation.

To Manipulate or Not to Manipulate

It's up to you. The controversy continues. A middle of the road approach might be to try chiropractic if nothing else is working after you've seen your medical doctor.

On the other side if you see a chiropractor first and get treatments, follow up with a visit to your GP or specialist medical doctor to be sure you have all of the medical bases covered including those that the chiropractor can't evaluate.

Some Warning Signs Of A Poor to Bad Chiropractor:

$ If he insists on taking X-rays of your full spine.

$ If he fails to take a complete medical history and do a clinical examination before beginning treatment.

$ If he claims the treatment will improve your immune function or cure a disease.

$ If he offers a variety of "vitamin cures" or "homeopathic" remedies.

79

$ If he tries to get other family members to begin treatments with him.
$ If he insists that you sign a contract for long-term care.
$ If he promises to prevent disease through regular checkups or manipulation. If he promises to prevent back pain through regular treatments.
$ If he suggests that chiropractic can be viewed as a primary health care function.

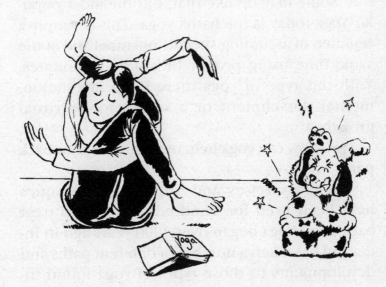

CHAPTER FIVE:
TREATING SCIATICA—
MORE NON-TRADITIONALS

YOGA

Many people have heard of Yoga but have no real idea what it is all about. Some think of it as a mystical excursion into an incense laden room with a long bearded guru smiling and meditating with them.

Some may be like that, but the most popular Yoga today is the hatha yoga. This is simply a regimen of assuming specific postures and at the same time using proper breathing techniques. With this type of yoga there is no meditation, mental detachment or a search for spiritual growth.

So how can yoga help us with sciatica or back pain?

Yoga exercises and breathing techniques have been used for hundreds of years to treat back pain. Yoga began over 4000 years ago in India and has taken a number of different paths and developments to those types of yoga found today. Other types include raja, tantra and jana yoga that do work with meditation and spiritual growth.

The yoga teacher usually works closely with each student on an individual basis to help correct any posture problems. Yoga has a system of postures called asanas. To go with this the teacher will work with the student to develop breath control which is called pranayama.

Many people have problems because they slouch too much and lose the unity of the body structure. Many back problems can result from poor posture, stress and structural imbalances.

Yoga enthusiasts say that learning even the simplest postures can teach people to see how they distribute their weight, how they use or abuse their spines, and show up any weak points they have in general posture.

The breathing aspect is a little more difficult for people to understand. Yoga teaches that there is a direct connection between people's emotions and how they breathe. Feelings such as hatred, fear, grief even anger can cause physical tension as well as emotional upsets.

By practicing proper breathing techniques while doing the proper posture exercises, a yoga student can learn to have some control over how his or her emotions affect the physical side.

Now, what about that back pain.

In yoga the spine is the center of the body, and all postural exercises focus on the spine. The biggest emphasis is lengthening the spine and re-aligning it. After this has been accomplished through the postures and correct breathing, a lot of a person's back pains will simply go away.

By aligning, the yoga people mean that the human body is in a straight line as if a plumb line were placed on the shoulder and the line would go through the hips and into the ankles in a straight line.

So far we haven't said anything that yoga can do to help out your sciatica. True. Part of the reason you have that herniated or pushed out disc could be your poor posture over the years. The benefit here is that after the disc is healed and the pain gone, you can take up this form of yoga to help keep your back from causing you any more trouble.

In many regimens today, flexibility is considered equally important for the back as exercises that promote strength. With increased flexibility and range of movements, a person can maintain better posture and help avoid all kinds of back problems.

HYPNOSIS

Can hypnosis help you with your sciatica pain? The answer is a cautious "it can" but it all depends on you—the one hurting.

Hypnosis comes from the Greek word *hypnos,* meaning to sleep. Most hypnotists these days say that hypnotism is a sleeplike condition physically induced in which the subject loses consciousness but responds with certain limitations to the suggestions of the hypnotist.

You've heard about the night club hypnotist who puts unsuspecting guests under hypnosis and then suggests that they do outrageous and embarrassing things on signal after they come out of their trance. This is not the kind of hypnosis we're talking about. Experts say people will not do anything under hypnosis that they wouldn't want to do without the hypnosis and will do nothing against their personal code of ethics.

Some experts say that hypnosis is when a person is in an altered state of awareness when the subject focuses on one subject and screens out all the rest. This lets the one hypnotized to get in touch with his or her subconscious and utilize it to help work out problems or control conditions.

One professional in the field says that hypnotism is only an acceleration of a natural tendency that we all have: the ability to screen out background noises and situations when we are totally concentrating on one idea, or project. For example a student cramming for a test might not hear the telephone ringing right beside him or her on the desk.

One of the goals of hypnotism for a sciatica pain patient is to help the patient to change the way the pain is perceived and how it is responded to. If the pain can be labeled as "background" to the patient, it will help him or her to downgrade it and screen it out. Then they can go about other activities without the hurt of the background sciatica.

Hypnotism does not cure sciatica.

Hypnotism can't repair or heal a damaged disc.

Hypnotism can't make your back pain go away.

However, hypnotism for many people can do more to relieve sciatic pain and other back pains than a bottle full of pain pills.

So, every time your sciatica kicks up with a thunderbolt of pain do you tear down to your hypnotist for a session? You could, but that would soon make you dependent on your hypnotist and run up your bills.

Most hypnotists say there is nothing difficult for a person to learn how to hypnotize themselves. It is a process that can easily be learned and then with practice a person can go "under" in ten to fifteen seconds.

Don't worry about getting "stuck" in a hypnotic trance. You've seen hypnotists bring subjects out of a trance in movies or on the stage. A person can come out of a trance by himself quickly and easily just by wanting to, or giving a self time limit of three or four minutes.

One man said he used self hypnosis at home and when others were around and he was "under" he wouldn't hear the telephone. He knew they were there and would pick it up. However, if he was alone and the phone rang, he would wake up at once and answer it.

Today a large number of dentists use hypnotism instead of Novocain for dental work. The patients like it and there are no vicious, painful needles to worry about. There have been cases where people have been operated on with only hypnosis as the anesthetic.

When hypnotism is used to help you fight your sciatica pain it's a form of mind over matter. You're convincing yourself that the pain isn't all that bad and that you can push it into the background and get on with your usual activities.

Hypnotherapy is regulated in most states where licensing is usually required. To be licensed certain standards and training are specified. Check your local telephone book yellow pages under hypnotism. If there are hypnotists advertised in your area, they are probably legal and legitimate.

HOMEOPATHY

This form of homeopathic medicine is not as popular as it once was in the United States, but proponents say it is growing rapidly worldwide.

The basic thrust here is that the patient is treated and not the disease. The homeopathic philosophy is that minute qualities of age old healing substances are used as medicine.

Natural remedies made from animal, vegetable and mineral substances are used and the entire group consists of about 600 medications. The average medical doctor has over 10,000 drugs to chose from.

Homeopathic medications have such small amounts of drugs in them such as belladonna made from the deadly nightshade plant, that they are non-toxic. Homeopathic medications are exempt from most of the Federal Drug Administration control since they contain such small amounts of drugs and medications. However if some homeopathic medication claims it can "cure cancer or AIDS" the FDA will pounce on them and make them prove it. Also, vague claims like, "for immune deficiency problems", will bring action by the FDA. For the most part the FDA has a hands off policy on homeopathic medications.

In the past, the homeopathic physician almost always prescribed one medicine at a time. This was because the remedy had been tested one at a time on humans, and there was no way to know how a combination of remedies would affect the patient. Now, however, many medicines for sale over the counter in health food stores and those that specialize in homeopathic medications, offer those with several ingredients.

One such is a medication for sciatica and neuralgia. It is said to be good for sciatica, neuralgia, rheumatic pains and backache.

The ingredients include: Belladonna (Nightshade)6X, Cimicfuga racemosa (Black Cohosh)6X, Gelsemium sempervirens (Yellow Jessamine)6X, Gnaphalium polycephalum (Everlasting)6X, 12X, 30X. Magnesia Phosphorica (Magnesium Phosphate) 6X, Spigelia (Pink Root)6X, and purified water. The mixture contains 20% alcohol.

The packaging for this medication goes on to state:

"Homeopathic Medicine is a safe treatment alternative for most minor ailments. Symptom relief is attained through stimulation of the natural healing process. Precise levels of homeopathic ingredients work safely and without side effects."

It says the medication is made "in accordance with the Homeopathic Pharmacopoeia of the United States."

Homeopathy goes by three principles:

1. **The law of similarities.** The idea here is that the patient's symptoms are studied carefully, and a medication is prescribed that exactly fits these symptoms. The idea is that a disease is cured by the same substance that causes the same

symptoms. Hippocrates wrote in 400 B.C. "Through the like, disease is produced and through the application of the like, it is cured." This is called the law of similarities.

2. The law of proving. This deals with the method of testing the remedies. A group of healthy persons is given a remedy. Some get placebo pills in a double blind test. The symptoms of each is carefully recorded. Those who got the remedy and have similar symptoms are written up in the Materia Medica book. This is the physicians reference book. If the symptoms are all the same, the remedy is then used to cure any sick person with the same symptoms.

3. The law of potentization. This refers to the way the remedies are prepared. They are made by a succession of dilutions and shakings and in some cases grinding, until the original substance has been diluted six times. The higher the dilution, the greater the potency.

CAN HOMEOPATHY TREAT SCIATICA?

A patient with sciatica came to her homeopathic doctor and described the terrible pain. The woman was pleasant and soft spoken and after some more talking with the patient, the doctor decided that a treatment called Colocynth, bitter apple, would cure her. The only symptom the woman wasn't showing was irritability and short temper.

The doctor let the woman wait for two hours and when she went back the patient yelled at her and scolded her for making her wait so long. The homeopath smiled and prescribed the cure she had chosen before. Now the last symptom of irritability had shown itself. The medicine worked and helped reduce the woman's pain.

Homeopathic medicines are extremely low priced compared to a regular pharmaceutical. A bottle of pills might cost $1.25 instead of $40 to $50 at your local drug store. Why? The five hundred to six hundred most used medications in the homeopathic medicine shelf have been there for the last one hundred and fifty years. Most are inexpensive to produce, none of them is patented, none is the result of a hundred million dollar research and development program at some huge pharmaceutical company. All are in the public domain. Neither is there a huge advertising budget to sell the drugs to the public or to the homeopathic practitioners which would be passed on to the consumer.

Lately in some areas there have been television advertisements for homeopathic drugs in general, but these are not promoting any single medication.

Homeopathic physicians say there is another difference between them and the allopath doctors. The homeopath spends much more time with their patients, getting to know them as individuals, sensing their moods and personalities as well as the problem they are having. They need to know this because often the mood of the patient is one of the symptoms of the ailment.

Will homeopathy help you get rid of your sciatica pain? It can't hurt. None of the homeopathic medications is toxic in any way. A child could gobble up a whole bottle of pills and suffer almost no bad effects. So, if it can't hurt, it might help.

OSTEOPATHY

Back in the late 1800's osteopathy was developed as basically a system of health care that highlighted the central role of the musculoskeletal system in health and disease and the use of spinal manipulation, the bending, twisting and stretching the spine, as a therapy.

Today the Dr. of Osteopathy, D.O., receives a scientific and medical training similar to M.D.'s, and in some states they function in hospitals and clinics and in private practice side by side with the M.D.'s. They generally take four years of college and four years of medical school and a year

92

of internship at an osteopathic hospital. They may go on to take additional training in fields such as rheumatology and orthopedic surgery, however most don't. About 90 percent of D.O.'s are in family practice.

Doctors of Osteopathy generally tend to use fewer drugs and less surgery and non-invasive methods as well as manipulation to help patients regain or maintain their health.

What About Osteopathic Doctors and Sciatica?

The D.O. will usually take a detailed history about the pain and the patient's past history. Then a palpatory examination is made. This is a gentle tactile use of his fingers to test the tissue tone and mobility around the pain area. A physical examination will be done and X-rays taken when necessary. The osteopath physician says this will enable him or her to either confirm or rule out the protruding or ruptured disc as the cause of the pain.

If it is a disc at fault, the D.O. will then use manipulative therapy to ease the pressure on the disc, then with gentle exercise and care, the slow repair can take place. In extreme cases surgery may be needed to remove any extruded pulp from the disc.

Back exercises and walking briskly on grassy ground or on a sandy beach is kinder to your back than running or jogging on concrete or asphalt roads or footpaths.

For help defining sciatica trouble, there are some reflex centers that doctors say look for considerable soreness. If they find it, this usually indicates a sciatica condition. These are at the front of the body and called ropy contractions which indicate lymphatic congestion associated with sciatic pain down one or both legs. These three points are:

◆ A ropy point that starts one-fifth the distance below the large bony protuberance of the upper leg bone and on for a distance of 50 to 90 millimeters downwards on the back outer part of the upper leg bone.

◆ A ropy point starting one fifth the distance above the knee and continuing upward for a matter of 50 millimeters on the back outer part of the upper leg bone.

◆ A ropy point in the mid-back area of the upper leg bone and one-third of the distance upward from the knee joint.

Osteopaths would rather have you prevent back trouble and sciatica than have to cure it. They have developed a given set of exercises for you to do to help insure good back health. These will be covered in the EXERCISE portion of the book in a later chapter.

State licenses and regulations vary from state to state concerning the practices of doctors of osteopathy. In some states they are on par with M.D.'s and work in and through hospitals and with insurance companies. In other states they are more restricted. Check for the availability and areas of operation in your state.

ORTHOPAEDIC PHYSICIANS

Don't confuse this group of M.D.'s with ortho-paedic *surgeons*. The orthopaedic physician is a specialist in soft tissue especially of the back. He works with injuries to the discs, muscles, liga-ments, tendons, joint capsules and other soft tis-sue of the back that can't be evaluated by X-rays or myelograms.

Orthopaedic medicine is the "nonsurgical management of soft tissue disorders of the mus-culoskeletal system. Surgery for ailments of the musculoskeletal system should remain within the domain of the orthopaedic surgeon."

How does this specialist find these non-bone problems such as a sciatica attack?

He uses a six major movement test: flexion, extension, right rotation, left rotation, right side flexion and left side flexion. First the patient does

95

each one by himself. Then the same motions are repeated but the patient remains passive, the muscles don't contract and the doctor can tell where the pain is coming from.

The last test is when the patient does the same motions against resistance which means the doctor can tell if there is pain, it's coming from a muscle or a tendon.

Usually if five or fewer of the motions result in pain, the doctors check for a protruding disc. This is not the extreme disc problem that ortho-paedic surgeons can find with a myelogram. These will be the smaller problems called a soft disc problem or a hard disc problem.

Many times the soft disc problem can be treated with traction. The hard disc type can often be cured with manipulation.

If these don't work and there is still pain, these orthopaedic physicians sometimes use a caudal epidural block. This is an injection of the anesthetic procaine into a specific spot in the back. It goes into the caudal aperture, a small opening in the tailbone. The procaine rises up the spinal canal to the lumbar disc level.

It works, but doctors aren't sure why. Some think that it desensitizes the nerve root and can also hydraulically separate a protruding disc from the nerve root or the dura mater which had caused the pain.

Sometimes one such treatment solves the sciatica or other back pain. Sometimes it might need to be redone every six months to a year.

Orthopaedic physicians are not in competition with orthopaedic surgeons. Actually they complement each other. If you're looking for an orthopaedic physician check with your local medical association.

WHAT ABOUT DIET AND SCIATICA?

Some dietary experts say there is a real help for sciatica sufferers when they pay more attention to what they eat.

Vitamin B complex and 500 mg of Vitamin C are touted as being a great help in reducing the pain of sciatica. One man said he had sciatica pain for 28 years. He said that his doctor put him on the above vitamin regimen and the pain went away.

An article in HEALTHY HEALING magazine extols the benefits of the following superfood therapy:

"Take a potassium broth every other day for a month to rebuild nerve health. Have a leafy green salad every day and a little white wine with dinner to relieve tension and nerve trauma.

"Eat calcium and magnesium rich foods such

as shellfish, tofu, whole grains, molasses, nuts and seeds, green vegetables. Take a good natural protein drink and drink mineral water. Avoid caffeine, refined sugars and chocolate."

Will it help? Can't hurt. You may want to give it a try.

Another source suggests these supplements to help your sciatica pain:

Calcium-Zinc-Magnesium tablets, four daily with vitamin D of 400 IU. Also B complex of 100 mg with extra B-1 of 100 mg, B-6 of 250 mg and niacin of 250 mg.

What about a full blown diet to help your sciatica? One has been recorded and it goes something like this:

The idea is to emphasize alkaline foods that should counteract the tissue acidity in your inflamed sciatica. Follow this closely:

Day One:
◆ Start with a glass of hot water mixed with the juice of half a lemon.
◆ For breakfast a glass of freshly made juice from apple, grape, carrot, orange or pineapple.
◆ Half way through the morning, take a glass of mineral water with a slice of lemon in it.
◆ Your lunch consists of only a glass of juice similar to what you had for breakfast. Make sure

it's fresh squeezed or blended.

◆ Break up your afternoon with another glass of water and that lemon slice.

◆ For dinner you get another glass of pure juice with a teaspoon of vegetable concentrate, yeast extract or concentrated apple juice.

Day Two:

◆ Repeat the menu for day one being careful to use only fresh juices sticking to the citrus. No bananas.

Day Three:

◆ As soon as you get up have a glass of fruit juice or hot cider vinegar and honey drink.

◆ Breakfast this day is fresh fruit salad with a quarter cup of sunflower seeds.

◆ For your midmorning pickup, try herbal tea, or a favorite juice.

◆ For lunch fix a raw salad from vegetables, and add a baked potato and baked onion. Add cheese or milled nuts.

◆ Afternoon break is for herbal tea.

◆ Dinner is a mixed raw salad or a mixed vegetable stew or broth.

◆ Before bedtime take another juice drink.

Days Four to Seven:

◆ Breakfast is a baked apple with raisins or fresh fruit.

◆ Break: herbal tea or fruit juice.
◆ Lunch: Raw salad with dressing, fresh fruit cup sprinkled with wheat germ.
◆ Dinner: Raw salad and dressing, vegetable broth, fresh fruit or baked apple or dried prunes.

This is not a diet for a big eater. If you have enough juice, give it a try. Remember, you said you'd do almost anything to cut down on that sciatica pain. So try the diet above. One good point. You're sure to lose weight over the week on all that juice and raw salads.

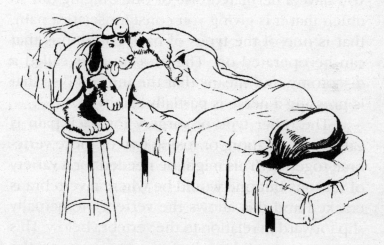

CHAPTER SIX:
TREATING SCIATICA WITH SURGERY

TO SURGERY OR NOT TO SURGERY?

A lot of people with sciatica and other back pain think that they can use the non-surgical remedies for as long as possible and when all else fails, they can always have back surgery.

Not true. There are many problems that can give you back pain, but only two that can be treated with surgery.

If an MRI or a CAT scan shows clearly that you have a herniated disc or one bulging out so much that it is giving you constant sciatica pain, that is one of the types of back conditions that can be operated on. The procedure is called a discotomy, and means that the injured disc that is pressing a nerve is partially removed.

The other type of surgery for back pain is called stabilization, or fusing two or more vertebrae together. This might be needed for a variety of reasons but one would be where a vertebra is cracked and this allows the vertebra to actually slip forward in relation to the vertebra below. This can cause terrible pain from pressure on the nerve roots. The problem is called spondylolisthesis.

These are the two major types of operations surgeons perform to help relieve back pain. There are a few other operations done for spine trauma, infection or a tumor, but an estimated ninety-five percent of all back operations are of these two types.

102

PROBABLY NO SURGERY FOR YOU

Today slightly more than ninety percent of all of you with back pain will never have surgery for it. You simply could not possibly be helped by such back surgery.

To be a good candidate for surgery your back pain must not respond to any other kind of treatment. Then it must be specific and the surgeon must be able to pin point the problem.

There is no way that even the best surgeon can help you if your back problems are caused by serious wear and tear of the spine and the discs over a long period of time.

DECOMPRESSION SURGERY

Surgeons call a discotomy one type of decompression surgery. This is the most common type and the offending disc is simply partially removed. Usually the doctor has to cut away a small portion of bone on the vertebra to be able to get to the herniated or bulging disc.

The surgery takes about an hour and starts with a two inch incision in the lower back. The surgeon pushes in and around the various muscles and ligaments. Usually there must be a piece of bone cut away to gain access to the problem disc. Doctors call this a laminectomy.

In a discotomy the whole disc is not removed. Once in the right place, the surgeon enlarges the existing hole in the disc's outer wall and scoops out most of the soft nucleus. This eliminates the pressure on the nerve and stops the pain. Then the surgeon moves the nerve root, ligaments and muscles back in place and stitches up the incision.

If a piece of bone is irritating a root nerve, it is located by X-ray and then removed much the same way that an offending disc is. The problem bone spur or growth is cut away relieving the pressure on the sciatic nerve root and the pain is eliminated.

SPINAL FUSION

The other type of surgery performed for sciatica or other back pain is called spinal fusion. This is when two or three vertebrae are fused together so they are motionless to give the back greater stability.

In about a quarter of the cases of decompression surgery, it is necessary to stabilize the affected area because the space between the vertebrae has worn down and is too narrow. This often means there has been too much wear and tear on the resident facet joints. To return the back to a more stable function, the surgeon decides that the fusion needs to take place.

Another time fusion is needed is when spondylolisthesis, the cracking and movement of a vertebra, does not get better with regular and conservative treatments. The cause of this problem is easy to see on an X-ray. Then fusing is needed.

FUSION SURGERY

The surgery begins much like that for a discotomy. The incision on the lumbar region is about three inches long because more space inside will be needed. First the surgeon will rough up the two facet joints, this will help them to heal better later and to fuse with new bone pieces.

Through another incision, the surgeon takes small strips of bone from the patient's pelvis. These bone strips are an inch long and less than one-sixteenth of an inch thick.

These bone sticks in effect become splints and braces that are packed by the surgeon against the damaged surfaces of the vertebrae. The body thinks the roughened areas have been broken and it rushes healing material to the site.

The effect is that the body fuses the roughed up vertebrae and the splints into a solid and stable unit, eliminating the pain and giving the spine more strength.

THE MICRODISCOTOMY

Gaining more and more favor is the micro-discotomy, which is simply the same discotomy but performed with a smaller incision and through a smaller area of the back with the aid of lights and a special operating type microscope. The benefits here are that the surgery takes less time, the incision is half the size as usual, there is less loss of blood, not so much after operation pain, a shorter hospitalization, quicker return to normal activities and less scar tissue.

While some orthopaedists frown on the smaller operating window and the procedure in general, many think that the micro type operation will be the accepted method in the future.

MAYBE NO OPERATION IS NEEDED

A recent newspaper headline said: "Can a $300 Injection Prevent a $10,000 Operation?"

The subject here is "chymopapain" an enzyme that is said to simply dissolve the offending nucleus of a herinated disc.

Does it work? If so why doesn't everyone use it?

Chymopapain has been a legally accepted drug in the U.S. since 1982. By now an estimated 50,000 doctors have taken courses and attended lectures to learn about the use of chymopapain. It's use is not as simple as it sounds.

Yes, it is invasive, but not nearly so much as even a microdiscotomy.

What kind of a patient should be considered for the use of chymopapain? One who has a herniated disc that is compressing a lumbar nerve root. Your typical sciatica sufferer. There should be a CAT scan or a myelogram to pin point a definite disc protrusion. Then the patient should have undergone up to twelve weeks of conservative treatments that have not produced any relief.

Not everyone agrees. Some orthopaedists say that if a patient has had severe sciatic pain for more than two years, a chymopapain injection isn't the best procedure. They say that after two years the spine has made adaptive changes, such as adhesions, that make the problem more complicated than just a herniated disc.

Many doctors report great success with the injections including long term relief. They point out that since there is no incision, there is no resulting scar tissue, which often leads to problems years later from discotomy patients.

For more information about doctors who use this injection treatment, contact:

Spinal Therapies Group
2215 Sanders Rd. Suite 500
Northbrook, IL 60602

HOW DOES IT WORK?

Someone said that chymopapain acts on the nucleus of a herniated disc the same way meat tenderizer does on a tough steak. The injected fluid breaks down the protein material in the nucleus of the disc, but doesn't damage the outer ring which is made up of cartilage. This means that the chymopapain dissolves the nucleus into a fluid that is absorbed by the blood stream and then excreted through the urine.

In effect it does the same job as that small scoop the surgeon uses to take out the nucleus in a discotomy. It does it slower but with no cutting of bone or tissue and is a thousand times less invasive.

THE PROCEDURE

It's done this way and it's relatively simple. Any orthopaedic surgeon who does diagnostic discogram tests or a radiologist should be able to do chymopapain injections with a little practice.

General anesthetic is used and usually the procedure is done in an operating room, although some surgeons prefer to use local anesthesia.

During the procedure the doctor is helped by X-rays shown on a fluoroscope screen so the needle can be positioned precisely. The doctor uses a six inch long needle and injects 1.55 cubic centimeters of chymopapain into the herniated disc's nucleus.

That's it. The needle is withdrawn and the patient goes into a recovery room. Recovery is about the same as for a discotomy. The sciatica pain is usually gone in two to three days.

Many orthopaedists think these injections are the wave of the future for herniated discs.

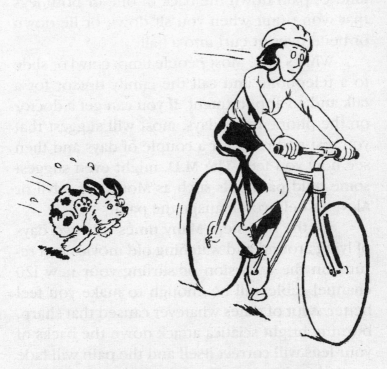

CHAPTER SEVEN:
SELF HELP THERAPY

FROM THE TOP

Let's get back to basics here. You have some back pain. This isn't that ache or mild discomfort you've felt before. Not just a few twinges, but a full blown scream-at-everybody-and-throw-things kind of pain down the back of one or both legs that won't quit when you sit down or lie down or bend over or curl into a ball.

What's first? Most people limp, crawl or slide to a telephone and call the family doctor for a talk and an appointment. If you can get a doctor on the phone these days, most will suggest that you rest and relax for a couple of days and then see how you feel. The M.D. might even suggest some mild pain pills such as Motrin or Advil or Aleve to help you manage the pain.

So, the first step. Many times this two days of lying around and watching old movies and re-runs on the television or surfing your new 120 channel cable will be enough to make you feel better. A lot of times whatever caused that sharp, burning bright sciatica attack down the backs of your legs will correct itself and the pain will fade away, then be gone. Yes, it happens.

All too often, though the pain won't go away and the Advil won't do the job.

You go see your doctor.

First he'll ask you a lot of questions, take a history of any back pain and get a physical exam of your back and legs and probably ask you to do some motions with arms and legs. When it's over he'll have a better idea what's causing your problem.

If he thinks it's sciatica, he still may give you some more pain pills and tell you to take it easy for another week, maybe two. Not bed rest but just no heavy lifting or unusual activity.

This is the conservative approach to see if the body can heal itself or if there is a problem that needs medical attention.

So, we come to the place where you can do some self help work to see if you can assist in getting your back in shape.

By now you know that if it's a serious herniated disc or a bad protrusion of the disc against a sciatic root nerve, a bunch of sluffing around and pain pills aren't going to cure you. But you can't be sure that's the diagnosis yet, so do what you can.

PAIN PILLS

These days pain pills come in all sorts of sizes, shapes and potency. Some pills that used to be prescription are now over the counter. Ibuprofen was a prescription pill for a long time. Now it's available in brand names such as Motrin and Advil and in many plain packaged house brands at major chain drug stores and grocery stores. Buy the house brand. Often they cost half as much as the name brand, and if they are 200 mg per pill, they will do exactly what the name brand will do

113

of the same potency. This way you aren't paying for the expensive advertising done by name brands.

Another fairly new former prescription pain pill is Aleve, the name brand which is naproxen sodium. This is tagged as a pain reliever and fever reducer and comes in at 220 mg for each tablet, but they claim 8 to l2 hours of relief for each two pill dose.

Other pills in this pain relieving category which are non-prescription and anti-inflammatory include good old aspirin, Anacin and Bufferin.

If you have long term pain and want a coated pill, you can get coated aspirin such as Entrophen, Novasen and Ecotrin. Here your stomach will not complain as it might on longer use of aspirin products. These all are non-prescription analgesic and anti-inflammatory.

If you can't take aspirin based pills or ibuprofen, try the acetaminophen non-prescription analgesics. These have no anti-inflammatory properties. They can't heal up any wounded tissue. They include Tylenol, Campain 500 and Atasol. Don't use these for more than ten days without consulting your physician.

On the other side of these come the prescription pills, many of them containing codeine.

114

These are not for you to be considering right now at this self help phase of your problem.

It might take a little experimenting to find the type of pain pill that works best for you. If you have a favorite for headache or some other pains, the same type of pill will probably work for you on your sciatica. It might help, but it might not.

HEAT AND COLD

The twins come into play here. If it's a recent problem, try the cold packs. This might be simply ice cubes in a plastic bag applied directly to your hurting back in the lower area. Be sure to put a cloth or towel between your back and the plastic covered ice cubes. You won't damage your skin that way. No more than about fifteen minutes at a time with the ice pack. The colder your back gets, the less active the pain nerves will be and you might slap down the pain for a time. You aren't curing yourself, just making the pain go away for a while.

A few days after the onset, you should go to heat. This can be dry heat such as with a heating pad, or damp heat with towels soaked in hot water and wrung out. Again don't let the too-hot towels be directly on the skin.

The hot pads will bring a flush of new blood

115

into the area. The added blood could bring in fighting white cells to help reduce any inflammation and start to repair tissue damage.

Again the hot packs should be used for no more than about twenty minutes at a time. Some say that by alternating hot and cold packs, you flush out the old blood and bring in a surge of new with the hot packs. If it feels good for you, do it.

REST YOUR BACK

Now what does that mean? Most doctors these days say that too much bed rest can be bad for your back. Where is the in between? If you did the two day slow and easy time after your first doctor call, you probably don't need to do it again. You still will probably spend a lot of time in a position that is comfortable for you. This might be lying on your side, sitting up, even standing.

The important idea here is not to go to work and don't do any lifting or bending to the side and lifting or anything like that which might further injure your already hurting back.

Common sense? That's the idea.

TRY THE NON-TRADITIONAL HELPS

Now is the time to take a shot at some of the non-traditional helps that some people say will cure your sciatica. Take a try at them and see. You've been to your M.D. who ruled out any deadly or ultra-serious disease or condition. Take a flyer, it might help.

See a Chiropractor. A lot of folks swear by their chiropractors. You've read about them in the chapter before. Hey, if a thirty or forty dollar first visit fee and evaluation and treatment is going to help your back, it will be worth it. The chances are that the chiropractor won't injure your back. He might do a manipulation and help out. Right now you're ready to try anything to stop the pain. Even if the pain is gone for only a day, it might be worth it for that small island of peace and quiet.

Try an Acupuncturist. Why not? Those little needles just might overload the major nerves and short stop the small nerves in your sciatica pain area from transmitting any pain. There is enough physical evidence that this works to give acupuncture some credibility. Remember, you have nothing to lose. Besides, those ultra thin needles don't really hurt.

What About Hypnosis? Read the section on hypnosis again. It just might fit you, might work for you. There are a lot of people out there who swear by hypnosis, the self-hypnosis kind, and they say it works, it helps them especially with pain. Hey, what do you have to lose?

Yoga And You. Yoga comes in all forms and shapes but the kind detailed in a former chapter might be something that you could do yourself to help strengthen your back and at the same time reduce your pain and your stress. Nobody says you have to get into the meditation end of things, the slow easy exercises and motions might be just what you need.

Biofeedback is Back. People are starting to take another look at biofeedback as a way to defeat pain, at least slow it down. The idea is not exactly self-help but it's something you can do without the aid of your doctor. Dig into it and check it out.

Acupressure? This is closely aligned with acupuncture. The main difference is the use of the thumb, fingers and hand for the pressure on the vital points, rather then the needles. It works for a lot of people, maybe it will work for you to help reduce your sciatica pain, even for a few hours. There is no way this can harm you.

Reflexology. Now this one is a little bit far out for most people, but there are thousands who swear by it. Massaging certain areas of the feet and hands just might have some effect on the rest of your body.

Homeopathy On The Homefront: Look

over the part previous about homeopathy. This is a do-it-yourself routine if there ever was one. Yes, there are professionals who can prescribe for you, but there are a lot of places where you can figure out things for yourself. The homeopathy medications are so mild and non-toxic that none of them can hurt you. There is one for sciatica mentioned above. Take a look for it in a health food store, and give it a try. What can it hurt? Hey the pills will be less expensive than no-brand aspirin.

How Well Are You Eating? Your lumbar spine is the end of the line for carrying the load of your upper body weight. The more it has to pack around, the more things can go wrong. Your weight might not be a factor in your back pain, but it could be. The odds are you'll have a healthier, less painful back if your spine has less weight to support.

Which is a round-about way of saying if you need to lose weight for your best body shape, now is the time to do it. Easy? Absolutely not. The only way, *THE ONLY WAY,* to lose weight is to take in less bodily fuel than you burn. Take in fewer calories, less fat and burn up more of both, and you lose weight.

There is no diet in the world that can do this—except the starvation diet which is not rec-

119

ommended. The best way to burn off fat and calories is with aerobic exercises. No, not the hard
driving stepping, dancing, jumping and jolting
you see on TV and in the gyms. Aerobic exercise
is any workout that is done on a continuous basis for twenty minutes or more.

The best is swimming, the next best is walking and a close third is bicycling. Walking is by
far the most convenient, takes the least special
equipment and can be done almost anywhere except in a car or in an airliner.

If you're overweight and out of shape, start
a walking program to go along with your exercising. The walking and your lower intake of fat and
calories will help you take off weight. The exercises will help strengthen and make more supple
your body's muscles. The combination is going
to help your back to get better and when it's well
help it to stay in better shape.

Don't sign up for a fancy diet. Don't buy specialty diet food. Simply read the labels and eat
no more than twenty-two to thirty-eight fat grams
a day if you're a woman. Men should not eat more
than twenty-eight to sixty grams of fat a day. The
higher total is for men doing active labor in their
daily jobs.

Read the labels on prepared food. It must
now list the calories and grams of fat. You'll be

surprised how quickly you can go over those totals. For example a breakfast of sausage, eggs and hashbrowns will kick in with thirty-four grams of fat. The average fast food hamburger will nail you with from forty-five to sixty grams of fat. A great three-quarter pound steak dinner with all the trimmings will set you back one hundred and sixty fat grams. You will have to concentrate on what you eat to keep your fat gram count down, but it will pay off.

The secret to losing weight: *EAT FEWER CALORIES AND GRAMS OF FAT THAN YOU BURN OFF EVERY DAY.*

THOSE FIRST FEW EXERCISES

There is a whole chapter on exercises later in the book. But right about now as your back is getting better, is the time to start with some gentle and easy exercises. We'll explain what they are and how they help later. But consider using some of them as you can.

For now the rule is: if it hurts, don't do it.

TAKE A SHOT AT WALKING

Why is walking so hot? As was stated above, walking is the easiest, least expensive, most adaptable and most do-anywhere do any-time aerobic workout you can do.

You can walk by yourself or with one or a dozen others. You can walk anytime of the day or night. You can vary the time you walk from one day to the next. You can walk faster or slower as the mood or your time slot or your energy level indicates. You can go a different route every day. You can go one mile one day and ten the next if you want to and if you can make it home without calling a taxi.

Walking has been around for a long time. It predates even the stair climbing machine and the workout gym. Walking gives your whole body a workout, your lungs, your legs, your back, your heart. Walking can also help to relieve the stress of everyday living, stress on the job or with the family and to improve your mood. It might even give you a better thinking process.

Walking can help you in a lot of ways, and it has no bad effects on your back.

Running? Yes, you get more calorie burning faster. However running on paving or blacktop or even a hard packed path can give your knees and your back a series of continual jolts each time your weight comes down on that one foot. Too many of these jolts, say running ten miles a day seven days a week, can do a lot of damage to cartilage in several parts of your body.

SWIMMING AND BICYCLING

Swimming has been described as the perfect exercise that works more of your body's muscles at the same time than any other workout. It also creates almost no stress on bones and cartilage by jolting, and will burn off one hundred forty-five calories in fifteen minutes of the crawl stroke. Only a six-minute mile run for fifteen minutes burns off more at two hundred sixty calories. Most of us can't run at a six minute mile pace for fifteen minutes. That's two and a half miles. Oh, if you run at an eight minute mile pace for fifteen minutes it will burn off two hundred fifteen calories.

For swimming you need a pool, lake, river or ocean to provide the water. Once you have that small problem solved, swimming is an excellent aerobic exercise that will help you burn off more fat grams and calories than you take in.

Bicycling at ten miles an hour on a level route will use up one hundred five calories in fifteen minutes. Not bad and does more than walking. Walking at four miles an hour for fifteen minutes uses up one hundred calories.

So, think about it. An aerobic workout will be good for you and for a stronger, less painful back.

WHAT ABOUT STRESS?

Some experts say that stress can be a big contributor to back pain. They say relieve your stress and you probably will help to relieve your back pain from sciatica or some other problem.

Stress is an emotional problem, not a physical one, but the emotions can often affect the physical in a powerful manner. Your back pain can actually help create your stress. This is magnified if you have a back pain or sciatica that is giving you fits for months.

Sciatica back pain can disturb your sleep at night causing extreme fatigue. It can affect your concentration on the job. If sciatica puts you out of work, this in itself can rag at your self respect, mean increased costs of care, chop off your income and quickly double up your stress quotient.

When you help generate stress with your back pain this in itself can make other problems worse: more unhappiness, more fatigue, more inactivity and these in turn produce more stress. It becomes a vicious circle of pain, stress and more pain.

How can you recognize stress in your life with sciatica pain? Stress affects almost everyone differently. It shows up in a wide variety of emotional and physical responses. Here are some common signs of stress. See if one or more of them fit your recent pattern of life:

◆ Feeling intense pressure on the job and at home.
◆ A feeling of being overwhelmed.
◆ Extreme impatience.
◆ Loss of interest in usually enjoyable activities.
◆ Muscle tension.
◆ Extreme nervousness.
◆ Withdrawing from usual activities.
◆ Problems with concentration.
◆ Low "flash point" of anger.
◆ Problems with sleeping.
◆ Trembling for no apparent reason.
◆ A sudden, radical change in appetite.

Are many of these symptoms of stress familiar to your recent way of life? If so, you probably are a victim of stress problems. How can you start to reduce your stress, which could also do a lot to help reduce your aggravated sciatica pain?

Try these methods:

◆ Start by taking a look at your life, your life style. Try writing down a list of what irritates you that leads to stress. Now look over the list and simply eliminate the stress creators that are not absolutely necessary to your life. For those you must do, try to relax and cope with them in a gentle, easy going way. It won't always work, but give it a try.

125

◆ Check local mental heath centers to see if there are any classes you can take on controlling stress. Often these are given at community centers and many are free.

◆ Read everything you can find on stress management. Often these books are available in your city library. Some are on tape. Also check your local bookstore for books and tapes on stress.

◆ If you have high blood pressure, anxiety attacks or headaches you think are brought on by stress, talk with your doctor about it. He may have some medications that will help, and some life style changes for you to put into practice.

◆ You may wish to investigate special programs such as biofeedback, that can help you with your stress levels. These are handled by a specialist in the biofeedback field.

◆ Your doctor may want to refer you to a specialist, such as a psychologist, who can advise you and work with you in special techniques to manage and lower your stress level.

IT'S A BIG SUBJECT

There is no chance that we can go into all of the ramifications of stress management here. It's a huge subject, complicated and with dozens of techniques and programs. Hundreds of books have been written on the subject.

What we want to do here is to remind you that stress plays a part in your sciatica pain, and that you need to be aware of it, and not to let it take over you life.

Realize that you are getting better, that the pain is moderating or will soon, and that you are doing everything you, your doctors and all the other helpers can do to cut off your pain at the pass.

Stress is a factor, but the more you know about it, and anticipate it, and move to short circuit it, the more you will be able to get back to your personal and more pleasant lifestyle.

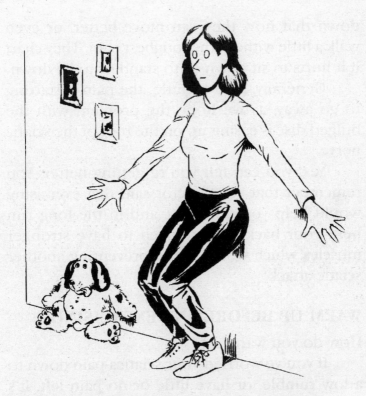

CHAPTER EIGHT:
YES, EXERCISE HELPS

So, let's say you've had a bad sciatic attack, maybe the first one, maybe not. You've seen the doctor and tried some of the self help ideas and guess what . . . you're getting better. Some people like to chart just how much better they are. They put down that now they can move better, or even walk a little without the toughest pain. They chart if it hurts to sit down or to stand or to lie down.

Generally, little by little, the pain is starting to go away, as we hope the problem with the bulged disc is easing up on the root of the sciatic nerve.

Yes, you can tell you're getting better. You remember that your doctor said that exercising would help you do better and in the long run help your back and stomach to have stronger muscles which would aid in preventing another sciatic attack.

WARM UP BEFORE ANY EXERCISING

How do you warm up?

If you've worried your sciatica pain down to a low rumble, or have little or no pain left, it's easier to warm up. Five minutes on a stationary bicycle or a five minute fast walk can get your body ready for your exercises.

For those of you who have considerable back pain but still want to do an exercise program, a fast walk warmup probably will do you more harm than good. If there still is pain, your best bet is to take a twenty minute hot shower. If you're water saving conscious you can do the same thing in a twenty minute hot bath, with frequent updating the hot water input.

The hot water warms up those major and minor body muscles and gets you ready for your workout. Now, even though your sciatica back pain hasn't all gone away, the hot water warm up will let you exercise to work on three benefits.

◆ Exercising will help stretch your lumbar spine area back to normal, which in itself is a benefit.

◆ Exercising can help your body become more flexible which will increase your normal range of movements.

◆ Exercising can help strengthen muscles that will help compensate for any lax ligaments which can't be tightened in your back.

EXERCISES DURING AND JUST AFTER A SCIATICA ATTACK

Much will depend on how much you hurt, how far along you are with your recovery and what the doctor told you to do. If you're in the two month "rehabilitation" period after an attack, you might not want to do any more exercising than a gentle walk around the house.

If you're past that stage, here are some gentle exercises and stretches that probably will work for you even though you still have some sciatica pain.

131

Remember the key word here:
If it hurts, stop doing it. . . .

WHAT EXERCISES CAN YOU DO NOW?

By this time you probably can walk around the house a little. This is a good time to move it outside and try to walk a block. If you can do that the first day you try it, do it for a week, then perhaps try a little longer walk. Walking is one of the best exercises for the body, despite what they say about the exercise machines and gadgets on TV. If the pain lets you, keep building up your walk until you can go a considerable distance without pain. Walking is an exercise? You bet.

If you don't want to walk, you might try one of the other good exercises for post sciatic patients. One is swimming. This again, can be done a little at a time, on your own schedule and as little or a lot as you can do. You are building up your muscles for your whole body, including your back. Here you will want to start slow and for a short time. It's another good way to get a start on an exercise program after sciatica. But, if it hurts, and it doesn't work for you, stop at once.

Oh, don't do the breast stroke, even if it is your best one. The breast stroke requires arching the spine sharply and this can irritate your already painful sciatica area. The breast stroke is

132

also bad for some people with specific kinds of back disease and pain. Check with your doctor to be sure. Generally, avoid the breast stroke and use one of the other resting strokes such as the side stroke.

AGAIN, IF IT HURTS, STOP

That's rule number one for doing any type of exercise especially after a sciatica attack. There are dozens of exercises that you can do that won't hurt. Do those.

The third easy exercise for those of you just coming off a sciatic attack is bicycling. Again, here you'll want to take it gently and easily at first, maybe only a block or two. If getting on and off the bike gives you lots of pain, this one isn't for you.

If you can work the bike do the usual build up of a little more each week until you are getting a good workout. As you go a little farther each time, you'll be building up your back and abdominal muscles and strengthening them which could help you avoid another sciatic attack.

EXERCISES FOR THOSE IN-BETWEEN TIMES

So now your back is feeling better, but it's not a

hundred percent yet. You need some in between exercises to help you get back in shape and strengthen your back and abs. Hail good fellow, follow along. That's what we're coming to right now.

STRETCH BEFORE ANY SERIOUS EXERCISING

Why should you stretch your muscles? If you've been to a competitive foot race, you've seen the runners doing a strange series of stretching exercises before they take their pre-race jogs. They know the value of warming muscles before launching an all out surge of muscle use in a tough half marathon.

The same idea applies to you. You need to get your muscles stretched out so they won't suddenly scream and yell at you as you go down in a heap.

For most of us, over the years, some of our ligaments stretch and sag. Other parts of our body may then contract and shorten to compensate. If there are any shortened muscles in your back or along your spine, they may be contributing to the reason for your back hurt in the first place. By stretching these out they will have the chance to get back in their proper position.

134

The First stretch:

Your hamstring muscles begin in your buttocks and go down the back of each leg and fasten to the back of your knees. When you stretch your hamstring, you will also be stretching your sciatic nerve. However if you're just recovering from sciatic pain or have had several bouts with it, you should stretch your hamstrings statically. This will not stretch your sciatic nerve and will not irritate the healing process.

EXERCISE: #1: Static Hamstring Stretch

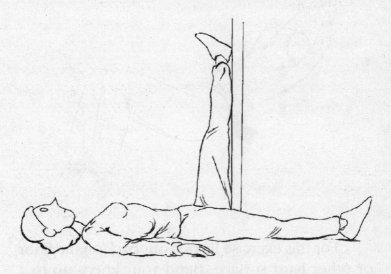

To do this stretch, lie on your back near a doorway. Move your buttocks next to the door jamb.

Extend your right leg through the doorway and the lift your left leg so it rests on the door jamb. Keep your leg straight. Move your buttocks forward until all of your leg touches the door jamb. Don't let your knee bend.

Hold the leg in position for twenty seconds. Relax. Repeat this process three times. Then change legs and flex the other leg for the three repetitions.

EXERCISE #2: The Pelvic Tilt

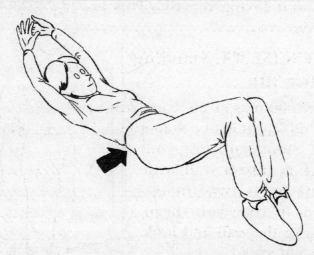

For this exercise lie on your back on the floor or other hard surface. Bend your knees up to a forty-five degree angle and keep your feet flat on the floor. Relax the muscles of your legs and feet.

Breathe normally. Press your lower back flat against the floor. Do this by tightening your abdominal muscles. This will make your hip joint roll toward your stomach. Hold this position for ten seconds and then relax. Repeat this procedure twenty-five times.

After you are comfortable with this stretch, try extending one leg to lie flat on the floor, all the while maintaining the pelvic tilt and with your lower back flat on the floor. Now bend the leg upward to the original position without losing the tilt. This is harder.

EXERCISE #3: Standing Pelvic Tilt:

After you master the lying pelvic tilt, try this one standing up. Stand and put your back against a wall with your heels two inches from it. Lean your head against the wall and look straight ahead.

Do the standing pelvic tilt by pushing your lower back toward the wall. Try to make your back as flat against the wall as you can and eliminate the hollow spot. Be sure not to hold your breath or tighten up your bottom. Press back for twenty seconds, then relax. Do this twenty times.

EXERCISE #4: The Low Back Stretcher:

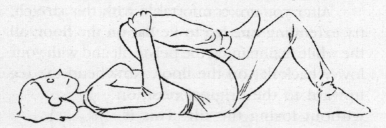

One of the basic stretch exercises on everyone's list. This is one that can relax your back muscles, ease tension, wipe out pains and aches in your shoulders and do a whole lot of good.

Do it this way: Lie on the floor with your head down. Move one leg to a forty-five degree angle with your foot on the floor. Lift the other leg up and pull it to your chest with both arms.

If there is pain due to a recent sciatica attack, bring your thigh as close to your chest as you can without any pain. As the pain lessens, bring your thigh closer and closer until it touches your chest. Hold it there for ten seconds, then return it to the bent knee position. Repeat this ten times on the first leg, the switch legs.

After you've stretched both legs, take a thirty second break, then lift both legs to your chest and tighten your arms. Hold for ten seconds. Do this double stretch ten times.

EXERCISE #5: Low Back Half Press Up Stretch/Rest Position:

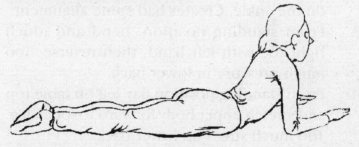

This is the single most important stretch/exercise in the book. It's not a half-pushup. It's the only tested and proven stretch to be done after a sciatica attack. It's an ideal flexor for the spine.

Lie on your stomach on a hard surface. Keep your hands, forearms and elbows flat on the surface. Lift your head and shoulders off the floor, keeping your elbows firmly on the surface. This gently arches your back. Hold for 10 seconds. Look straight ahead. Do a series of ten to fifteen of these to help relax your back. As you get more flexible, try straightening your arms.

HERE ARE ELEVEN STRETCHES *NOT* TO DO!!!!!

1. From sitting position, stretching head forward and resting it on your legs or ankles. Too much stress on your lower back.

2. From a standing position, lifting one leg to the rear and pulling upward with your hand on the ankle. Creates bad spine alignment.

3. From standing position, bend and touch right toe with left hand, then reverse. Too much pressure in lower back.

4. From standing position, lay leg on table top and stretch upper body forward to touch leg. Too much stress on lower back.

5. From standing position, bend over and touch toes or put hands flat on the floor. Over stress on lower back.

6. From prone position, stretching upper body upward on fully extended arms and arching head and neck backwards. Neck arch puts too much stress on upper neck and spine.

7. Sitting with legs crossed in lotus position and rounded back. Too much stress on lower back.

8. Sitting with one leg extended, other one to the side and stretching torso and head forward to touch extended leg. Bad for the lower back.

9. Rolling of the head too far to the back. Over-stretches the neck and upper spine.
10. Lying down, arms extended, lift legs over head and try to touch toes to floor behind head. Over stretches lower back.
11. A shoulder stand, with legs extended fully directly above shoulders. Serious pressure on upper neck bones.

NOW SOME STRENGTHENING EXERCISES FOR YOUR BACK

So, your back and legs are feeling better. Most or all of the pain of the sciatica is gone. You want something more to help keep your back in better shape so you don't run the risk of another sciatica attack. Good strengthening exercises can help. Here are a bunch that can be done without the use of weights. These are using the weight of your body itself to get the job done. A kinder, softer approach.

The warning here is that if you think you're ready for work to help make your back stronger, and you try some of these exercises and they hurt, **stop the exercise at once.** The rule is, if it hurts, don't do it.

EXERCISE #6: The Half Sit-Up:

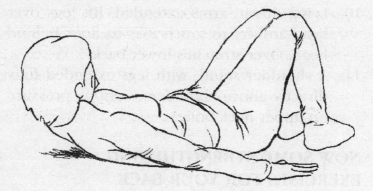

Some vital warnings about sit ups:

DO NOT DO FULL SIT-UPS WITH LEGS FLAT ON THE FLOOR AND COMING UP INTO A FULL SITTING POSITION. THIS IS DRAMATICALLY HARD ON YOUR LUMBAR SPINE AREA AND CAN CREATE OR MAKE WORSE ANY LUMBAR PROBLEMS THAT YOU HAVE. DON'T DO FULL SIT-UPS WITH YOUR TOES HOOKED UNDER A COUCH OR HAVING SOMEONE HOLD THEM. BAD FOR YOU.

This exercise is done to make your abdominals stronger. These half sit-ups are a good way to tighten up and make your abdominals flatter.

Do them this way:

Lie on the floor with your knees bent and feet flat. Rest your arms at your sides or on your abdomen. Tuck in your chin and push your arms forward and lift your head and shoulders off the floor. Don't go too high. Hold this position for ten seconds, then return your head and shoulders to the floor. This one will soon make your abdominals start to burn and hurt. Stop. The next time you'll be able to do more. Work up to twenty. Then if you want more, take a short break and do another set of twenty. These can't hurt your back and will help wonderfully well with your abdominals.

EXERCISE #7: Partial Leg Lift:

This workout will help strengthen muscles in your knees, abdomen and the front of your hip. If done correctly, they will also help you to keep your spine and pelvis stable when you move your legs which will help you

143

to sit and bend more properly.

Lying flat on the floor, place hands on each side of lower abdomen and help your lower back remain flat on the floor. Lift one leg to a seventy degree angle keeping your knee straight. Hold leg up for seven counts, then lower it to the floor. Don't let your trunk and pelvis move as you lift or lower your leg. Now repeat with the other leg. Do this exercise from seven to twenty-five times, depending on your strength.

EXERCISE #8: Half Squat Rotation:

This exercise is designed to work on getting more strength in your legs and to help improve your balance.

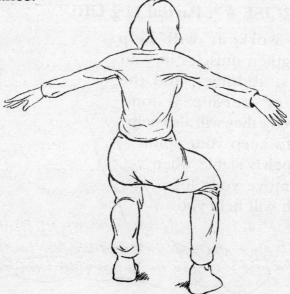

Begin standing with feet spread a little more than normal so they are directly under your shoulders. Do a half squat and hold it, then move slowly in a circular motion shifting your weight in a circle around your feet. At all times keep your trunk and head in a straight up position. You may want to use your arms as a counterbalance as you move around. Your legs will show strain first. Do for fifteen to twenty seconds. Stand and rest legs, then do two more repetitions.

EXERCISE #9: The Bridge:

Here you can work on strengthening your buttocks, back, thighs and abdominals. With practice it will help you to stand taller, to climb stairs easier, and to get up from a low chair without strain.

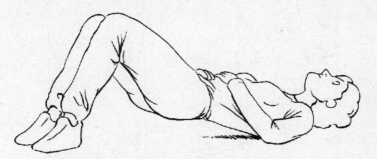

Lie on back with knees drawn up to forty-five degree angle. Slowly tighten lower abdominals and buttocks to flatten your lower back to the floor. Now lift your pelvis off the floor an inch or two at a time until your pelvis and low back come off the floor. Tighten your buttocks as you lift. This forms a bridge between your feet and your upper back and shoulders. Hold position for five seconds as you breathe normally.

Now lower your pelvis slowly an inch at a time until you again have your lower back flat on the floor. Do this exercise from seven to fifteen times.

EXERCISE #10: Leg Lifts While Standing:

By doing this exercise in a consistent manner, you can strengthen most of the major muscles in your legs. When you maintain good head, pelvis and trunk position during the workout, you will fur-

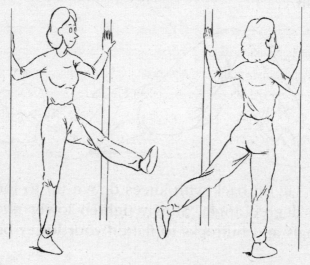

ther aid in maintaining a good posture. This one can also help with your balance and coordination.

Always use a desk or doorway for balance when doing these exercises. Hold your head and trunk in a good posture position.

Hold on to a doorway with both hands, keeping your head and trunk directly over your hips as you lift one straight leg forward as high as you can without moving your torso. Go only as high as you can comfortably. Hold the leg at height for eight seconds, then slowly lower it. Repeat ten to twenty times with each leg.

Now do much the same thing lifting the leg to the back. Lift as high as possible without changing your torso or head position and hold for eight seconds. Then lower leg slowly. Repeat with each leg each way for ten to twenty times.

EXERCISE #11: Abdominal Leg Extensions:

Helping to strengthen your abdominal muscles is an important part in healing sciatica problems as well as other back hurts. Your abdominal muscles are what support your spine and pelvis from both sides and the front. Since these muscles are so active in supporting the spine, they must be worked smoothly, with no straining, jerking or high speed repetitions. This is one of a number of abdominal workouts you can do.

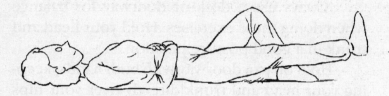

Start lying on your back with both knees in bent up position. Slowly push out your right leg until it is straight and six inches off the floor. Keep your back and abdomen straight and back flat on floor. Hold leg off floor three to five seconds, then pull it back slowly bending your knee and placing foot on floor in bent knee position. This is a hard one. Do three to five times on one leg, then switch to the other leg.

When you can hold each leg off the floor for ten to fifteen seconds for ten reps, try the same thing only with both legs at the same time. This one is for advanced exercisers only.

EXERCISE #12: Hand And Foot Extensions

You've probably never heard of your extensor muscles along your back which are in your buttocks, thighs shoulders and neck. These are the

148

muscles that hold your spine stable and help you maintain your balance. This hand and foot extension exercise will help strengthen these muscles and help keep your spine straight and strong.

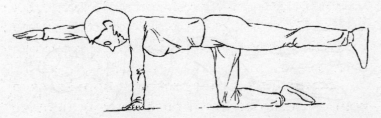

Get on the floor on your hands and knees and keep your back straight and your head and neck in line with your back. Move your weight to your right knee, lift your left leg and fully extend it backwards keeping it level with the floor. At the same time shift your weight to your left hand and fully extend your right arm forward keeping it parallel with the floor.

Hold the position for three to seven seconds. Return both hand and foot to the floor. Repeat this action seven to twelve times on each side.

EXERCISE #13: On The Side Workout

These exercises from lying on your side help toughen muscles that give stability for your lower back, hips and pelvis. They help to hold your back in good posture.

149

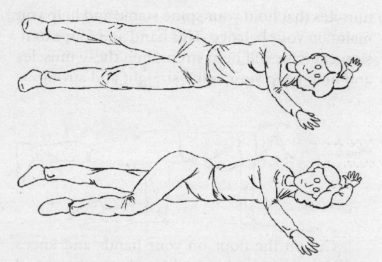

Lie on the side with your head on a pillow or on your bent arm. Your top arm extends in front to the floor for balance so you won't roll forward. Your legs rest on top of each other. Now rotate your top leg upward, keeping your knee straight to about eighteen inches off the floor. Hold that position for three to seven seconds, then slowly return it to its original position. Repeat this twelve to twenty times.

Now move your top leg forward with bent knee and put it on the floor freeing the bottom leg. Lift the bottom leg off the floor as far as comfortable and hold for three to seven seconds then slowly return it to the floor. Repeat this twelve to twenty times.

EXERCISE #14: Leg Lift Balance:

This simple exercise will help to train your abdominal and back muscles to lengthen and support your spine as well as help with your basic balance. Stand with your feet about a foot apart. Stand tall as you tighten your lower abdominal muscles. As you keep them tight, lift one knee waist high and hold it there for five seconds. Use your hands at first if you need to, to maintain your balance.

After five seconds, lower leg and lift the other one for five seconds. Do each leg ten times alternating.

EXERCISE #15: Side Bends

This is another easy exercise that can help limber up your back and at the same time strengthen your side torso muscles. It's good to help you get back into the harder exercises and your normal work patterns.

Stand with your feet about eighteen inches apart. Reach your right arm down toward your knee and at the same time lift your left arm over

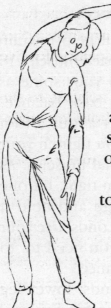

your head and bend it as far to the right as you can. This will also bend your head, shoulders and torso to the right.

Return left arm to your side and do the same thing on your left side stretching with your right arm over your head.

Do this on each side from five to ten times.

EXERCISE #16: Spine Rotation:

The idea here is to limber up your spine. Spinal rotation is required in many daily activities. This is a good way to keep your spine ready for a work or play activity where the rotation is needed.

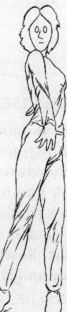

Stand with your feet about sixteen inches apart, hold arms away from body to side at about a forty-five degree angle. Rotate your torso and head to the left as if looking back over your shoulder. As you do this let your right heel come off the floor. Tighten your lower abdo-minals to support your lower back. This twisting motion will help your whole spine to do a gentle rotation. Hold this position for five seconds, return to the start.

Now do the same maneuver twisting to the right as if looking over your right shoulder. Again, hold for five seconds.

Repeat this from five to ten times on each side.

EXERCISE #17: The Resting Clam:

If your lower back starts to feel tired or tight, this is a good exercise to help loosen it up and to rest.

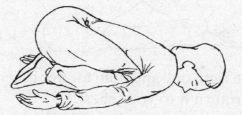

Sit on your legs as in the picture, bend forward with your chest against your thighs and lower your head to the floor, then extend your arms back along your legs.

Achieve this position slowly. It will come easier with practice. When you can do the position fully, maintain it for fifteen to thirty seconds, then lift up and relax. Do this position for three to five times depending on how you feel.

EXERCISE #18: Leg Thruster:

Start by lying on your back with both knees pulled to your chest. Then hold left knee and extend right leg to ninety degree vertical position keeping your foot flat on top. (Don't point your toe upward.)

Hold this position for five to ten seconds until you feel a stretch in the back of your leg. Return right leg to chest.

Now hold your right leg and extend your left leg upward as you did the right one and hold for five to ten seconds. Then return it to your chest.

Repeat this exercise on both sides from five to ten times.

EXERCISE #19: Gentle Abs Workout:

Here is an easy abdominal exercise that can be done from hard to easy to suit your needs. Do as many and as with as much lean as fits your needs —and your muscular development.

Sit on the floor with your knees bent at a forty-five degree angle, your torso is held erect

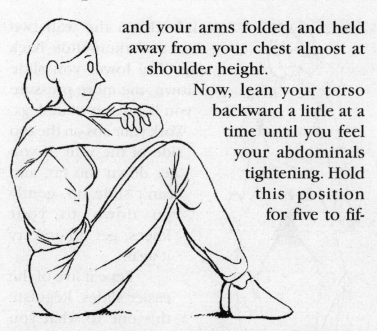

and your arms folded and held away from your chest almost at shoulder height.

Now, lean your torso backward a little at a time until you feel your abdominals tightening. Hold this position for five to fif-

teen seconds while continuing to sit tall. Look straight ahead during this lean. Then return to the starting position. Repeat this exercise from five to ten times.

EXERCISE #20: Holding Up The Wall:

This exercise can be a killer if you go too low on the wall. It then will exercise your legs more than your torso, but it's good for both. Adjust the depth to which you go for your desired workout and for which area.

Easy does it here. Stand with your back against a wall and your arms at your sides. Slowly

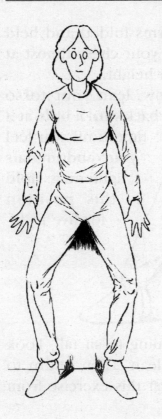

slide down the wall two feet and then slide back up. The lower you slide down, the more pressure you'll put on your legs. Work your abs on the top side of the wall. If you get down too far, and can't slide up, gently go down to your knees, get up and try it again.

Repeat five of the easier slides. Regulate this one to what you want it to accomplish. Excellent for leg strengthening as well.

EXERCISE #21: Chair Bend Down:

For a general back stretch that won't kill you, try this chair bend down. Work it on each side and hold as long as you feel comfortable.

Sit on a chair for this one and bend forward so your chest is touching your knees. Extend both arms and lean to the right so you can put your clasped hands outside your right foot. Hold five

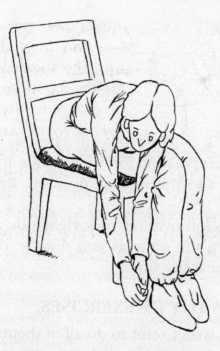

seconds. Return to upright position. Now bend forward and lean to the left and put clasped hands outside your left foot. Repeat on each side from five to ten times.

EXERCISE #22: The Sidewinder Slide:

The sidewinder will help work your abs and your leg muscles as well. Remember to slide, not lift your leg.

Lie on your left side with knees and hips slightly bent. Cushion your head on your folded arm. Now slide your right leg upward until you

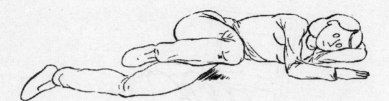

can bring it as close to your chest as possible. Hold in that position for five seconds and slide it back down to the starting position. Repeat five times.

Then roll over on your right side and slide the left leg the same as you did the right one. Again, repeat five times.

THAT'S A LOT OF EXERCISES.

True. You won't want to do all of them. Pick out the ones that seem to help you the most. Use some of the flexors and the stretching ones, then dig into the others and find out which ones help your back, and which ones you need most to strengthen your back so you won't have any more sciatica attacks.

Remember, moderation in exercising, especially when you start out. Don't forget the cardinal rule in exercising to help your back:

If it hurts, don't do it!

158

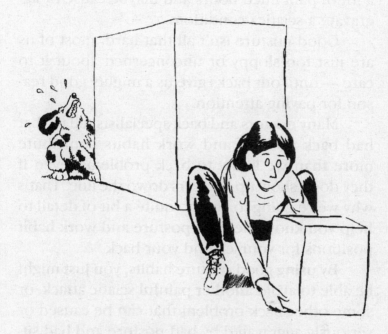

CHAPTER NINE:
Sitting, Standing, Bending Back Tips!

Let's just admit it at the outset: Most of us don't know a thing about good posture, good sitting or standing posture, or even how to sit at a desk, a keyboard or a work table so our back is not thrown out of kilter and getting ready to give us a lot of pain filled hours and maybe cause or aggravate a sciatica condition.

Good posture isn't all that hard, most of us are just too sloppy or unconcerned about it to care — until our backs give us a mighty good reason for paying attention.

Many doctors and back specialists tell us that bad back posture and work habits contribute more than we know to back problems, even if they don't show up for years down the line. That's why we're going to go into quite a bit of detail to help you know the right posture and work habit positions for yourself and your back.

By using good posture habits, you just might be able to avoid another painful sciatic attack, or some other back problem that can be caused or seriously aggravated by bad posture and bad sitting, standing, reaching and lifting habits.

SITTING

Most of the experts agree that just sitting in a chair or on a couch is one of the most stressful positions you can get into in relation to your low back and neck. Millions of people spend most of their day sitting down at a desk or computer terminal during their working day. Millions more spend a lot of time in arm chairs and kitchen chairs during the day at home.

Some Bad Sitting Problems

Crossing Your Legs

When you cross your legs while sitting, you tip your pelvis to one side and this produces a curve in your spine. Usually this curve is temporary and will go away when you stand or move to a new position. The best way to counteract this sideways curve is to alternate your leg positions. Cross your right leg over your left the first time, then a short time later reverse the cross which reverses the spinal curve and negates any long term problem.

Here you won't be in any trouble unless you consistently and without fail cross your legs always in the same manner. Another tip is to push your pelvis firmly against the chair's back before you cross your legs. This will give you stable platform.

Stressful Sitting

Don't sit in such a position that you must tighten muscles in your back or your neck just to maintain your position. Don't lean forward in your car when driving, stressing the muscles in your back. Try not to tense up the muscles in your shoulders and back when doing that final report at your desk or pounding out a letter or a pro-

161

posal on your keyboard. You may be able to check yourself on this type of stressful sitting by noticing if you are grimacing while trying to sit tall, or frowning or even straining the muscles at the front of your shoulders and your neck.

Instead push your hips against the back of a firm chair, lean back, relax and let the chair hold you in a good sitting position.

Don't Sit In The Same Place Too Long.

In sales training there is an axiom: The mind can absorb only as much as the seat of the pants can stand. The idea was that people in meetings for over 50 minutes should be given a "seventh inning break" by standing and talking or just looking around.

We humans are not designed to sit in one position for hours at a time. Sitting is much more stressful on the spine than standing. Even in a good sitting position, it's good to give the body a break and get up and move about or change your sitting position. Cross your legs the other way, move to a different chair, do some work that requires you to be standing for a time. Work out a variety of sitting positions to keep your body in better tune.

The Famous Sitting Slump.

In a sitting slump your back is rounded, your

162

tailbone tends to roll under your hips and your head is thrust forward. This position often occurs when you sit on a chair or sofa that is too soft, with a poor backrest or one too far from the front of the sofa, or the back is too concave or sometimes too low. Best solution, avoid this type of seating.

What does this position do to your spine? Your spine is unnaturally curved from front to the back of the chair and then outward toward your hips. Your neck is arched backward and your head is thrusting forward in front of your shoulders and chest instead of being positioned above your spine. If you sit this way for any length of time, or on a regular basis day after day, your spine can develop strange curves and your head and neck can give you a lot of problems.

This position can also increase compression and over stretching of the pelvis and lower back. The slump position is often the culprit in much of the low back pain that patients feel. This pain can be in the lower back or neck. It also can mean problems in breathing since the diaphragm can't work correctly and your ribs don't have room to expand as they normally do.

Constant sitting in this position for a long time will mean you probably will have trouble standing up straight when you get up to walk.

Other problems include headaches from sitting too long in this position as well as related pains in the neck and shoulders.

Now Some Good Sitting Ideas

If you have to sit down for long periods, learn a variety of ways to sit comfortably and with good posture.

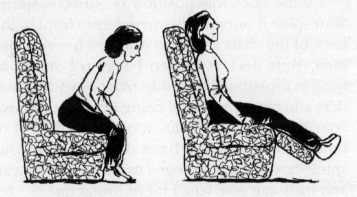

One of the basics for good sitting down is to know where your pelvis is in relation to your chair. Most people sit down in a chair about in the middle of the seat. Once landed you need to move your pelvis to the rear so it contacts the back of the chair.

To do this put your hands on the arms of the chair or the seat and lean forward and lift yourself up a few inches and shift your pelvis backward until it touches the back of the chair. Now lean backward to the back of the chair and you have a perfect sitting position. Your head, neck and spine are all in an arrow straight alignment.

If you have a reclining seat in your car on the passenger's side, it's an ideal way to relax while maintaining good posture. Push your pelvis on the front part of the seat, then lean back with your legs out fairly straight. You'll have good posture with your head and neck and spine all in alignment.

On a regular chair you might try sitting forward more. Do this by positioning your pelvis against the back of the chair, then lean forward to get nearer to work or eating or even driving. This way you can still keep your head and neck and spine in a straight line with no slumping.

You might try the same thing as above, only move to the front edge of your chair with your pelvis. Then leaning forward with your head, neck and spine in a straight line, you get a different type of sitting down yet in good posture.

You've probably heard about lumbar supports. These devices are used to help support the lower back area to maintain the natural curve of your back.

These pillow type devices come in various sizes and shapes so you might need to experiment to find one that fits you just right. You'll want to be sure your posture is right before you test for a support. Keep your pelvis against the back of your office or work chair, then check how you feel. If you still need some lower back support, test with a rolled up magazine or a towel to get an idea of what size support you need.

Positioning the lumbar support is by trial and error. Once you find the right spot, you may wish to tie or tape the support against the back of your chair. That way it won't slip or fall out and it will be there everytime you sit down.

Okay, you've been sitting there an hour, you still have a pile of work to do and can't go for a ten minute walk. What's to do?

Some body movements can help you relax and still let you keep working. Try these :

◆ Rocking your pelvis. Rock your pelvis and low back forward and up so your tailbone lifts off the seat and your low back will arch forward. Help this by using your hands on the chair arm to lift an inch off the chair. Hold the position for three to five seconds and repeat it four times. Then get back to work.

◆ If you do a lot of reading at a desk, try using a slant board that will lift the material three to six inches off your desk and make it easier to read. This will help eliminate a head down position that can be murder on your neck and spine.

◆ After sitting a long time, try doing your reading or writing job at a makeshift stand up desk. Sometimes a file cabinet is the right height. If it's too tall, use a small wooden box or a foot stool. Twenty minutes there and you're ready for your desk again. Some novelists work all day at specially designed stand up desks, writing with pens or computers. It works.

◆ Try propping up your head with your elbow on your desk and your palm under your chin. You can still write and read, but now the muscles around your neck have support and can relax and your head still stays upright.

YOUR STANDING POSTURE

All of us can stand, but are we standing in a good posture, one that supports the body in a balanced position and uses little muscle energy to do it? That's the main thrust of good standing posture. Good standing posture: Looking at a standing figure from the side, there should be a straight line from the ear, down through the body, through the middle of the leg and to the foot. No forward thrust of the chest or the buttocks pushed out to the rear. Fairly simple.

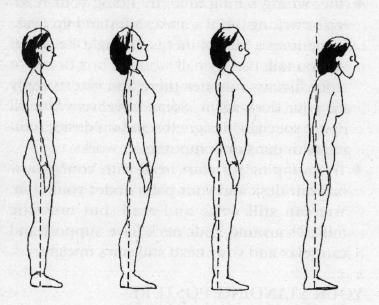

Always doing it is tougher.

Correct standing puts less pressure on your spine than sitting down or a variety of other movements. Try to keep it that way with good posture.

Standing tall is a term many physical therapists use to urge their patients to pull in their stomachs, pull in their buttocks and get a more straight line posture.

If you have a stand up job such as washing dishes or working at a bench, it's a good idea to have a foot stool nearby so you can lift one foot on the stool. After a few minutes change the foot on the stool. Also if it's a one handed job, leaning on one arm can also help to reduce the strain on your spine.

If you have a long standing situation, simply leaning back against a wall or counter will help support your body and also assist decompressing your spine. Yes, that's good.

Another help for long term standing is to do a sway. Simply shift your weight slightly from one foot to the other or rock forward onto your toes and then back to your heels. This will help to reduce some of the strain on your back from standing

The Leaning Crane Problem

Some people have a forward leaning standing posture. This puts a lot of strain on your body. Here your knees are pushed backwards until they lock in place. This tends to tip the pelvic and low back area to tilt forward and increase the back's arch. This can also push down the chest bringing the head and neck into a forward and dropping down position.

It's extremely stressful on body muscles to stand in this position even for a short time. It feels like you're going to fall over forward so your body muscles pull back and keep you standing.

Solve this problem this way: First unlock your knees, let them go forward so they bend ever so slightly and so they are directly above your ankles. Your new knee position will help you level your pelvis so it is better aligned over your legs. Lift your chest and take a deep breath so it is aligned over your pelvis. Lift your head and straighten your neck so you have the straight line from your ear right down your spine and through your pelvis and down your leg.

By standing this way you'll take a lot of strain off your lower back and at the same time reduce muscle use and tension.

The Slump Stand

Some people have a rounded back when standing with their head thrust forward. This comes about by tilting their pelvis outward and excessive bending of the knees to throw everything out of that straight alignment.

Take care of the problem this way: Bring your knees back to a normal position, not locked but not too bent. Straighten back your shoulders and your neck and head to stand tall. Then your chest will come up and your rounded back will be gone. You'll be standing with that straight line down your side from head to ankle.

WHAT ABOUT LIFTING AND BENDING OVER?

Lots of ways you can hurt your back and maybe bring on or bring back a case of sciatica by lifting things the wrong way. Let's show some wrong ways and right ways to do the job.

1. To lift something off the floor, squat in front of it with your knees wide, keeping your back straight, pick up the item, then using your legs, come upright with the pressure of the rise on your legs. Keep your back straight at all times. You may squat either with your feet flat on the floor, or on your toes, whichever way is best for you.
2. When bending down or squatting, keep your feet wider apart than your shoulders to give yourself a good working foundation.
3. If you're leaning forward to do a task, as taking clothes out of a front load dryer, lean one hand or arm on the top of the dryer and extend one leg behind you to help keep your spine straight as you work.
4. If carrying suitcases or packages, balance your load on each side for equal stressing. If this is not possible, change hands with the load to balance out the stress.

171

5. When reaching or lifting something over your head, keep your body alignment true to reduce the strain. Always use a step stool to avoid overhead lifting if possible.
6. When picking something up from the floor, do the baseball squat with knees bent and arms resting on your knees. Go down easily and pick up the light object, then push off knees with your hands to stand.

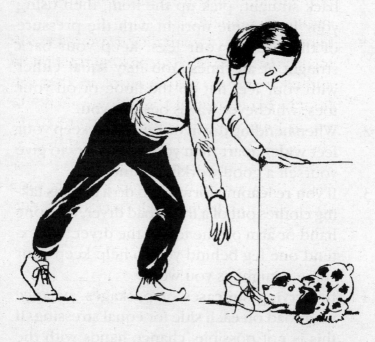

7. Do the crane bend to pick up something near a table or chair. Rest one hand on the

chair, extend one leg out behind you keeping your spine and back straight, bend down and pick up the item, then push up with your hand and return the stretched leg to a standing position.

8. Half kneeling bend is good for working on or near the floor. Bend down with one knee on the floor, the other knee bent. Especially good if your back still hurts. Keep your back perfectly straight during this move and there should be no pain.

9. Squatting is not a good idea if you are working on the floor, such as picking up a lot of spilled items, or scrubbing or waxing the floor by hand. Instead of squatting, get down on all fours and then use one hand to do the work with the other hand helping to brace your body. This is the easiest on your back. Even sitting down and bending over to do work on the floor will excessively strain your back.

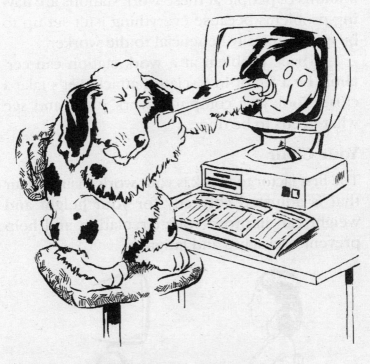

CHAPTER TEN:
SCIATIC PROBLEMS IN THE WORKPLACE

A COMPUTER WORK STATION

First let's look at a typical work station for a computer. Millions of people these days spend most of the day in front of a keyboard to a computer.

175

Millions of people at these work stations are having problems because everything isn't set up to be ergonomically beneficial to the worker.

A back problem at a work station can certainly be a factor in a sciatica attack. Let's take a closer look at a computer work place and see what needs to be done.

Your Chair

The first factor to check is your work chair. A chair that is adjusted correctly for your height and weight can improve your circulation and help prevent backaches and fatigue.

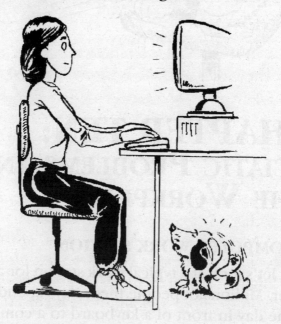

Sit in your work chair and move your hips against the back, then straighten up in your usual work position. Are you comfortable? Can you reach your keyboard and other items that you need in your working day? Does the backrest fit snugly against your back? If it does not, you should adjust the backrest until your lower back is supported fully.

If your chair does not have an adjustable back rest, try to get one that does. If you can't, you may need to use a small pillow or rolled up towel against the back of the chair to help support your back properly.

Chair Height

Is your chair adjusted for the right height for you? The right level of your chair will help relieve cramping and stiffness in your legs as well as stress and tension in your shoulders and neck.

Sit in your usual manner in your chair and place your fingers on the home keys of your keyboard. Your forearms should be parallel to the floor. If they are not, lower or raise your chair to a level that allows your arms to be level.

Now check your foot positions. Move your feet forward until your knees are at a ninety degree angle or slightly more. Now your feet should be flat on the floor and about six inches of room between your stomach and they edge of the keyboard. You should also have three inches or so of room between your legs and the bottom of the keyboard platform.

Your Work Area

Your whole work area should be arranged so you can reach everything without any strain on your back, neck or shoulders.

Start by checking your computer monitor, your screen. When you are seated in your properly adjusted chair, the top border of your screen should be level with your line of sight when you look straight ahead.

If the screen is too low, raise it with a magazine or telephone book or a block of wood under it exactly the right size. If it is too high, you may have trouble lowering it. This is because many screens sit on top of the computer or on an electrical union box and electrical surge protector. In this case you might need to lift your keyboard and raise your chair height to compensate. At all costs get your screen at the right height.

Screen Distance

Now take a look at the distance your eyes are from the screen. This may depend on your eyesight and the focal length of your glasses or your contacts. Some people get special glasses that have the exact focal length needed for the way the operator likes to sit at the computer. This can be anywhere from eighteen to thirty inches. An adjustment is easy to make here, simply move the monitor and screen forward or backward until it is at the right distance for your eyes and your lenses.

We talked about the keyboard before in relation to your arms. Your forearms should be level with the floor when you're working. This takes into account that your wrists are also straight, and extension from your arms that are also straight.

Some keyboards have adjustments for height on the back of them. Adjust as needed. Some can be raised so they are slightly slanted. Many typists like this factor and use it. More keyboards being made now have a wrist rest built into them. This gives the lower part of your hand a convenient place to rest when not actually working to help reduce wrist strain.

Some of the new keyboards are split down the middle and set at a gentle angle with the keys angled backward away from the operator. These are said to be ergonomically easier on the worker. Try them to see. They will take a minor adjustment. Many people love them.

Another important item for the computer work station is the placement and height of your document holder you will be working from. Be sure it is as high as the screen and as close to the screen as possible. This prevents moving your head and neck up and down to pick up copy from the bottom of a page eight inches below the bottom of the screen.

Workplace Lighting

Be sure there is no glare on your screen from either inside or outside light. If there is a window in your room, place your computer screen at right angles to it, or facing it, so no glare can interfere with easy reading.

If there is overhead lighting or a desk lamp, be sure that they don't glare off your screen. Adjust them so they are parallel or just behind your screen. Never let a desk lamp shine directly on the screen.

Try a Minibreak

Working at a computer all day can be tiring. Give yourself a two minute minibreak every hour or so. One easy way is to lean on your elbows placed on your desk. Cover your eyes with your cupped hands shutting out all light. Stay in the dark for a minute or so, then slowly remove your hands.

If your shoulders start cramping or hurting, try this. Raise your hands beside your head and then squeeze your shoulder blades. You'll feel the pull. Hold for five seconds and do it three to five times. Another good one is to shrug your shoulders as high as you can. Try to lift your shoulders up to your ears. You might hear some joints popping. That's good. Do the shrugging three times, then relax. Your shoulder hurt should be gone.

Another one is to sit in your chair and drop your arms outside of the arm rests. Now shake your hands or spin them for a few seconds. Stop and relax, then do the exercise three times.

For really bad cramping shoulders while working at a desk or computer, lie on the floor and pull one leg to your chest and hold it for ten seconds. Then do the other leg. After five reps on each side, pull both legs up and hold them for five seconds. You might want to do this in a private room, but the relaxing effect on your shoulders is remarkable.

That's the advice from experts on your work station, and how to be in your office at a desk and still not have back problems or any back strains that could lead to a sciatica attack.

Heavy Work Situations

If you're a laborer or one who must do heavy

work much of the day, learn how to get the work done without hurting your back. A few helps:

◆ If something has to be lifted, get some help.

◆ Usually it's better to push a heavy object rather than try to pull it. Simple mechanics.

◆ If you do heavy work, many states now require that you use a support belt. You've seen them in stores around the country. While not a cure all, they can help support vital areas of your back under stressful lifting situations. Still maintain good lifting practices.

◆ Know your limitations. If a job is too hard for you, don't be afraid to ask for help or to be reassigned. Many firms are well aware of back problems, and the cost of such injuries on their workmen's compensation insurance rates. Management will probably work with you.

◆ Don't do any lifting or pushing that you think might bring on a sciatic attack.

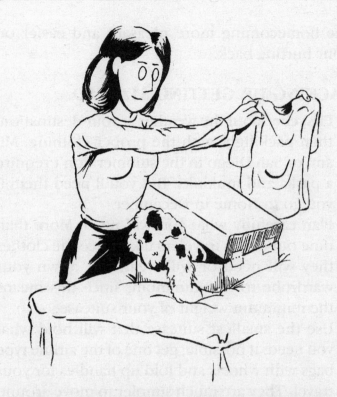

CHAPTER ELEVEN:
TRAVEL, SLEEP, SEX AND CHORES

Just because you have a bad back is no sign you stop enjoying life, and this means you'll want to do some traveling. Here are some ideas and helps to make that getting ready to travel, the trip and the homecoming more pleasant and easier on your hurting back.

PACKING UP, GETTING STARTED

◆ First check out the weather at your destination, then pack light with the proper clothing. Miami or San Diego in the summer don't require a parka and mukluks. But you'll need them if you go to Nome in December.

◆ Plan carefully what you will need. More than nine out of ten travelers take twice the clothes they will need or will wear. Cut down your wardrobe to the minimum, since this means the minimum weight of your suitcase.

◆ Use the smallest suitcase that will hold what you need. If possible, get one of the airline type bags with wheels and fold up handles for your travel. They are much simpler to move around an airport or motel or hotel lobby.

◆ Pack your suitcase on a bed. It's much better than bending over to the floor. Remember to take along emergency gear such as a heating pad and cold packs that can be frozen— just in case you need them.

◆ Use extreme caution putting in and taking luggage out of a car trunk. Try not to bend forward and lift the luggage with no support. Move it slowly if you must do this. Better yet, pay a red cap or porter to unload your trunk and get your luggage to a check in window or curbside check station if flying.

◆ If no manpower is available, use a rental or free luggage cart available in most airports and train stations.

◆ If you do strain your back with luggage or from stress, try to get an ice pack on the affected area as soon as possible. Many airports have first aid stations that will help you. Stretching out while using the ice is best.

◆ Wear durable, safe walking shoes for travel. Fashion is not a factor here. Many well dressed people wear athletic shoes for traveling for their comfort and the shoe's strength and no slip qualities. Forget high heeled shoes or those with flimsy sides or mushy soles.

◆ If you must unload luggage from your trunk. Put one foot on the bumper or in the trunk

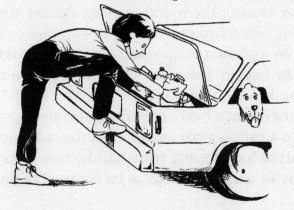

itself. This helps support your back during the lift where the weight is primarily on one foot, then on the other one.

◆ Use the half kneeling position to pick up a heavy bag. Remember to change hands if you have only one bag and must move it any great distance.

◆ Traveling by train, plane or car is going to mean a lot of sitting. Use the various sitting positions we talked about before to stay comfortable. On a plane ask for two pillows to use for back and neck support. There are usually lots of pillows available. If you're on a train or in your car, bring along a favorite pillow or two for the same use.

◆ Take a break. When you're driving a car or truck, be sure to stop for five minutes every hour for a break. Walk around your car, take a brisk trot a block away and back. Rest your eyes by closing them and leaning against your car for two minutes.

◆ On a plane take a stand up break, walking to the back of the plane or to the bathroom. Just make sure you don't get run over by the flight attendant's beverage cart in the aisle.

◆ In a car, as a passenger, lean the seat back and stretch out with your hands high over your head. Push your legs as far forward as possible and stretch as tall as you can. This can relieve a lot of pressure on your spine.

SLEEPING WITH A HURTING BACK

A lot of people with a sciatica back hate to go to bed at night because it's going to mean another night of increased back pain and little if any sleep and lots of turning and tossing and staring at the night light and the lighted clock which seems to be running at about half its normal speed.

Problems

Let's take a look at what could be part of the problem: the foundation. What kind of a mattress do you have? Generally speaking, the experts say that a firm mattress is best for those of us with hurting backs. Why? A firm surface will tend to keep your spine from flexing as it does when your body sags into a soft mattress. That flexing can cause you pain and anguish and not allow you a whole lot of sleep.

To the basics: Find out if a firm mattress is best for your back. Take six or eight thick blankets and lay them on the floor and sleep on them for a night or two. How did it go? Did your back feel better there than on the mattress you're now using? If it did, a harder mattress is probably needed.

187

Want to make one yourself? Easy. Pitch out your mattress and spring set, or at least stand it up in the garage for possible later use. Now if you have a wooden bed frame use that. If you don't have a good bed frame get nine eighteen inch high concrete blocks and stand them on end three on each side of your new bed and three down the center. Now get a half inch plywood board. They come four feet wide by eight feet long, and set it on the blocks. At a specialty store, buy a chunk of foam rubber six inches thick and the size of your bed board. You might have to stitch or glue pieces together to make it fit. Now put on your mattress pad and sheets and blankets and try out your new bed.

This will be a firm type mattress.

Another way to firm up a bed is to put a 3/8 inch thick piece of plywood between your mattress and your box springs. One nice thing about this is that on a queen or king sized bed, this board can go on your side and not bother your non-hurting back spouse. The board will give you a much firmer feel to the mattress without the expense of buying a new one.

Give this a try for a week or so and see if it makes any difference. If it doesn't, your next move should be to go to a store   and lie down on a variety of harder mattresses. Stay on the one you like for a half hour or more and see if your back responds. If so, you might have found your new mattress.

Sleeping Time

What about the physicality of sleeping?

Start out before you go to bed. Oh, the best way to get the best sleep is to go to bed the same time every night and get up the same time every morning. This way you program your brain and your system into a routine that will help you get to sleep normally.

Another tip. You probably should have a resting position for when you first hit the old sack, then a sleeping position. For example you might lie on your back when you first get to bed, then after ten or fifteen minutes of relaxing and cooling out, you turn on your side and tuck one arm under your pillow and in ten or fifteen seconds you drop off to sleep.

Now, what about the best sleeping habits for the bad back person?

If you've been working hard all day and are still tense and tight at bed time, try some relaxing and stretching moves to start to wind down. Some simple hands over the head stretches, or some side bends and "shaking out" your hands and legs will usually be enough. Don't do any hard exercises, such as one hundred pushups just before bedtime. This will elevate your heart rate and put your nervous system on "special alert" that might not let you get to sleep for hours.

Now, you're relaxed, you've had your ten minutes of "resting position" in bed, and you're ready for sleep. What's the best position for your bad back?

Most bad back people say that unsupported stomach lying is hard on the back and can aggravate any sciatica or back pain.

The clue here is "unsupported". A pillow often can turn a bad sleeping position into an ideal one.

Find the best pillow for you. If it's under your head when you lie on your back, it should be full enough so your head can lie to establish that "straight line" between head, neck and spine. Your head shouldn't fall backward or be propped too high. Either one will put a strain on your neck and spine. On your back you'll also need to put pillows under your lower thighs and legs.

Now, most of us do a lot of turning while we're asleep, so how can you use a pillow when you might be on your side a half hour after you get to sleep and then on your stomach an hour later? It's a problem. Usually the pillows work best to help you get to sleep. After that unless the position is too extreme, it probably won't wake you up even when it's hurting your back a little.

One easy solution to helping but not totally solving this situation, is to put a lumbar roll around your waist. This will help fill in the void when you lie down. What's a lumbar roll? They are sold commercially, or you can make one yourself.

Take a bath towel and fold it in half lengthwise. Then roll it tightly from the side so you have a roll about three feet long. Adjust the length so it will fit snugly around your waist. It could be two to three inches thick. Now fasten it securely with safety pins so it won't slide around as you change positions at night.

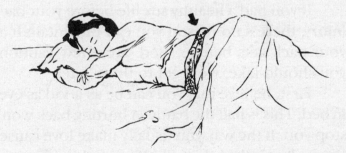

This is good for lying on your side or your back. Try it for a night or two and see if it helps your hurting back.

The whole idea is to get a good night's sleep

without having to use any of the over the counter or prescription sleeping aids. This way is the best way.

Whatever position works best for you, try always to keep your head, neck and spine in good alignment. That's part of the key to a good night's sleep.

BE SEXY EVEN WITH A HURTING BACK

Yes, don't worry, a hurting sciatica back doesn't have to slow down your active sex life. In fact, some of the suggestions here might make your sexual gratification even better.

"Not tonight, honey, I've got a damn back ache again."

Hey, it doesn't have to be so.

If you had a healthy sex life before your back injury, there's no reason you can't maintain it as your back gets better. There are a few cautions you should take, we'll get to those later.

First, believe that you can be as good as ever in bed. This is half the battle. A hurting back won't stop you. If the way you usually make love causes you only a little pain and it's something you can live with, there's no reason you should change your positions or your tactics. On the other hand, if your usual positions give you so much pain you can't continue, then it's time to look for the new

192

positions we'll talk about soon.

Second, if you do need to make some changes, talk it over with your spouse. A loving partner will be ready and willing to make adjustments that will help continue your good sexual experiences. Be direct, clear and make it plain that a little adjustment now will make things better for both of you.

Third. You might even get creative and come up with some new ways to achieve mutually satisfying sexual experiences even without coitus. Think about it. Manual and oral stimulation are two of the most obvious, but get creative.

Fourth. If you must make some changes, get agreement with your spouse about what needs to be done and how to do it. This is a partnership situation and both of you must be in agreement.

A Backache Kind of Lover

So, what's next? What will hurt and what won't?

If your lovemaking is working and not painful in spite of your hurting back or your sciatica, go right on in the same pattern. You may want to try something different just for variety even so, and the positions shown here will be safe for most people with back pains.

◆ In any position, avoid an extreme swayback. This serious arching will hurt your spine and if you have sciatica or other spine related problem, it's bound to cause you fits of pain. Keep your spine straight or slightly bent forward during intercourse.

◆ Never bend forward with your knees straight, not even if you are in a lying position. This puts a great deal of force on your lumbar spinal area. It also stretches your sciatic nerve and you don't need this since it's already a problem. You can curve your spine forward a little, as long as your knees are bent.

◆ Don't use positions like lying flat on your back or on your stomach with your hips extended out straight. This includes the famous missionary position. This position will stress and stretch your psoas muscles that run from the front of your spine to just below your hip. This muscle helps control a woman's vaginal contractions.

◆ Whenever you can, use a position so your hips are flexed, it will help to avoid irritating your lower back.

Now what positions are best for bad back people?

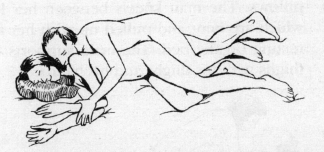

1. This is the best position for either partner with back pain. The partners are lying on their sides. The male is behind in a close spoon fashion Neither has to support the weight of the other one. The woman must be careful about getting a swayback position here. This one is the best even if you have a serious backache and protracted pain. This one won't increase that pain.

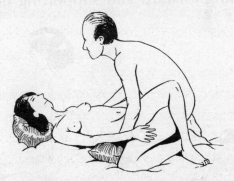

2. Good for the woman with back pain. She lies on her back with upper torso supported with

195

pillows. The man kneels between her legs which are bent and pulled up with her feet resting on the bed. The male supports her thighs with his thighs and his hands.

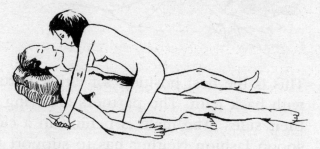

3. Another one good for the woman with a painful back. The man lies on his back with his feet spread. The woman kneels on top with her hips flexed. She must avoid swayback by leaning forward and supporting her shoul-

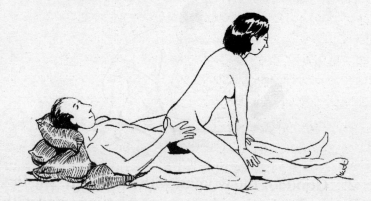

ders with her hands near his shoulders. The man's head and torso should be lifted with a few pillows to slightly flex his spine. This is also a good position for the man with a hurting back.

4. Similar to the one above with man on his back with head and torso supported by pillows. Woman kneels at his waist but faces his feet. Woman can support her body with her hands on his thighs or knees or on the bed. She should be careful not to irritate the man's back with too much pressure on his knees.

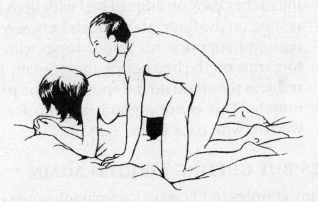

5. This position is good for the male's backache. Woman is on all fours, man kneels behind her resting his weight on his hands on the bed at her sides. His back should be slightly rounded.

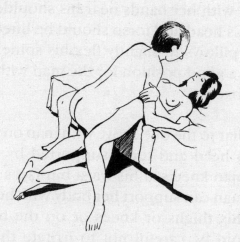

6. Good for the male's hurt back. Woman is ly-
    ing on her back on edge of bed with both feet
    resting on the floor. Male kneels between her
    legs and supports his upper torso with his
    forearms on the bed beside the woman. This
    reduces the strain on the spine and the psoas
    muscle. This is not a good position for the
    woman with back pain.

YES BUT GETTING STARTED AGAIN

Many couples hold off on lovemaking when one
or the other has a serious back problem. Good
idea. But when the partner is on the mend, when
the pain is controllable, when the urge is there
and the back isn't all that bad, take a try.

Use the best method for the first time, probably the spoon position shown above. It just might work, and if so, that will be one more step in getting you back to normal.

If one of these positions doesn't work, try some of those other innovative methods we talked about that can give satisfaction without actual intercourse.

HOUSEHOLD AND YARD WORK

Here are some more tips for taking care of your sciatic back when you do ordinary jobs around your house, yard and garden. Most of these regular activities mean you do a lot of lifting, bending and make repetitive movements such as raking leaves. You've done these things for years. Maybe a quick review of them will help you do them so your back will feel better. By doing them the best way you will certainly keep your sciatic back from feeling any worse.

Outside The House

◆ You have a garden. It needs planting. The onion seedlings are waiting for you, all 120 of them in that small pack. You've spaded the ground and it's ready. How to get those thin little shoots safely planted without killing your back.

199

Don't stoop over to do the job. Get a cushion or drop cloth to kneel on, then reach forward with your back straight and dig your furrow and lay the onions in carefully an inch apart. Still keeping your back straight you won't put any undue strain on your spine. Fill in the small furrow and sit back and wait for them to grow.

You might also kneel on one knee and keep the other foot on the ground and your knee at your chest. You can even lean on your upper thigh for more support. Now plant as before.

A third way is to kneel down with one leg behind you and sit back on that leg keeping your other one bent so your knee is ready for resting on as you lean forward and do your planting.

Sitting down and reaching forward usually doesn't work very well from a space and reach standpoint, and it is often straining on your back.

If you are a gardener, don't be afraid to get down in the dirt. You'll do better with your plants and help save your back at the same time.

◆ If you rake up your leaves in the fall, try doing it this way. Set your feet two feet apart and keep your whole body lined up in front. Now reach your rake out to your left or right and rake directly in front of your feet. As that area is cleaned, step forward and take another swath. This keeps your body from bending and twist-

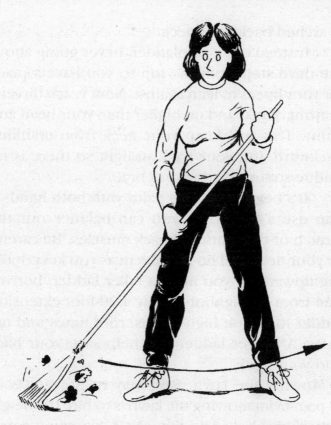

ing and gets the yard cleaned quicker.

Don't stand with your feet close together and rake at your side. This means a lot of unnatural twisting and pressuring all the wrong points.

◆ Painting? It can be a disaster for your back, unless you do it right. Reaching high and standing on tip toes to reach that one last spot can put a lot of stress on your sway back and your arched backward neck.

Instead use a stepladder, never going above the third step from the top so you have a place for your knees to lean against. Now, reach directly in front of you and no higher than your head and paint. This will keep your neck from cranking backward and your back straight so there is no undue strain on your vertebrae.

It's best to learn to paint with both hands if you use a brush, so you can balance out the stretch of the arms and back muscles. Be careful or your neck will be a problem as you keep looking upward. If you need a taller ladder, borrow one from a neighbor or buy a 20-foot extension ladder for those high places, roof times and tall trees. A longer ladder will help save your back and your neck.

◆ Mowing the lawn. Best way to prevent back pain from mowing the lawn is to hire the neighborhood kid to do the job. If that won't work, try this: Always use gloves if a gas engine mower vibrates too much through your hands and irritates your back. The gloves will help. Wrapping the mower handles with foam rubber and taping it on will help even more.

Always try to keep your back straight, arms extended and straight and walking upright when pushing a lawn mower. Don't drop into the arched back problem or the swayback. Concentrate on keeping your hips in and your back straight and eye looking straight ahead. Oh, watch where you're moving as well.

◆ Shoveling Snow. If you live in one of the cold weather states, shoveling snow comes as one of the undeniable privileges of home ownership. Hire the kid next door is best, but if this

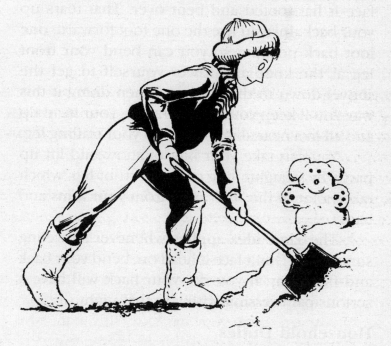

doesn't work, be sure to take all the precautions available.

Wait a day for the sun to do the job.

203

When this doesn't work, get out a shovel. Try not to use the huge grain shovel with a scoop two feet wide. A smaller shovel might be better.

Shoveling snow or dirt or gravel is one of the worst things you can do for your back. Shoveling simply puts a tremendous strain on your back. If shovel you must, try it this way.

First you have to get down to the snow. Don't face it flat footed and bent over. That tears up your back. Instead use the one foot forward, one foot back position so you can bend your front leg at the knee and lower yourself to get the shovel down to the ground. When doing it this way you'll keep your back straight, your head up and all in a near alignment with your trailing leg.

You can take your bite of snow and lift up partly by straightening out your front leg, which takes a lot of the "lift" away from your arms and back.

The same idea applies whenever shoveling something. Don't face it head on, bend your back and flail away. If you do, your back will have a serious pain session with you that night.

Household Duties

◆ The Old Vacuum Cleaner . . . This doesn't have to be a disaster for your back, even a hurting sciatic back. Don't bend your back and lean forward as if you're in a motorcycle race. Your back will kill you. On the other hand, don't over arch your back trying to stand tall and bending over at the same time to reach the vacuum handle.

Best way is to take the fencing type stance, with one foot forward and one back. Your forward knee can be slightly bent. One hand on the vacuum handle is enough. Now use the other hand on your bent knee for added support. Keep your pelvis level and you'll do the vacuuming in record time and not feel it. Oh, for even less strain, change hands on the handle half the time. Evens up the load. For best balance keep your right foot forward when your left hand is on the vacuum. With your right hand on the vacuum handle, put your left foot forward.

If you have to clean under a table or furniture, it often works well to go down on one knee with your other leg bent in a half kneel. This lets you work under the furniture without over stressing your back.

◆ Taking laundry out of a dryer is a bend over situation when it's a front loader. Instead of bending and rounding your back, try putting one leg out behind and leaning on the top of the dryer with one hand and removing the dry clothes with the other. This way your back will stay fairly straight and relieve any pressure on your spine. Then when carrying the hamper, be sure to pick it up from a squat and lift with your legs.

◆ If you wash dishes by hand at your house, try this. Before starting, open the cupboard door below the sink. As you start washing, lift one foot up and put it on the four inch raised bottom of that cupboard. This will help level your pelvis and reduce strain. You may also want to tense your buttock muscles and push your pelvis level and firmly against the counter.

◆ The backbreaker: making the bed. Never an easy or quick job, the bedmaking can be tough on backs. Avoid slumping or arching your back when you bed make. One good way is to drop a pillow at the corner of the bed, kneel on it and smooth out the sheets and blankets while kneeling. It makes it a lot easier, you're in a good position to do the job and it's a lot less of a strain on your back.

PREGNANCY AND YOUR SCIATICA

As you know, pregnancy causes a lot of changes in a woman's body. One of them is the physical shifting of the spine to accommodate the change in the center of gravity of the woman and the increased "front load" of an advanced pregnancy.

To give a woman a chance to maintain her balance, the spine must accept much more weight than normal along with the related stress on the vertebrae and the associated ligaments and muscles.

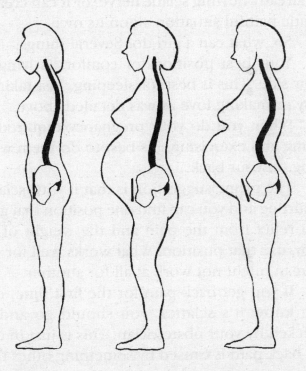

Adding to this structural problem comes the hormones. One is released during pregnancy to relax and loosen the pelvic ligaments. This is so on birth day the baby's head can move through the birth canal easier. The big problem is that this hormone, relaxin, also loosens up the sacroiliac and other joints the same general area which can cause you more problems.

So, pregnancy does create some new problems for the spinal column. It can further irritate an already hurting sciatic nerve, or it can create a sciatic painful situation all on its own.

So, what can a girl do? Several things.

Your best position for comfort is lying on your side. This is best for sleeping, just taking it easy or making love as was detailed above.

When you do your pregnancy required relaxing and exercising, it's best to do them while lying on your back.

The prime suggestion is that if your sciatica is hurting and you can find one position that gives you relief from the pain and the weight of the baby, use that position. What works well for one woman might not work at all for another.

If you get back pain for the first time, or if you know it's sciatica, you should go and be checked by your obstetrician. This is just in case the back pain is caused by something other than your pregnancy or the sciatica. X-rays are prohibited during your first four or five months, depending on your doctor. If no new problems are found, stick to your exercise program and get relief from the sciatica as your doctor prescribes.

Remember, you're pregnant, so the doctor won't be giving you any serious pain medication. If the pain is too great, you might ask your doctor about a kind of corset designed for pregnant women to help reduce back pain. Heat and massage sometimes do wonders, including that long soak in a warm tub of water. You'll be continuing your regular program of swimming, walking or biking. One great benefit . . . the whole thing can't last more than nine months.

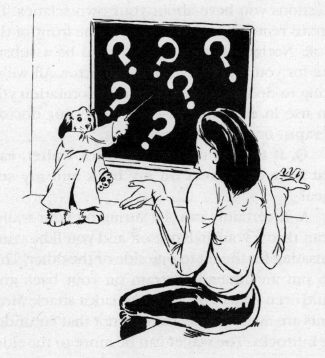

CHAPTER TWELVE:
QUESTIONS ABOUT
YOUR SCIATICA

If you don't ask—you'll never find out. Here are a group of questions that many people with sciatica and back problems ask their doctors and therapists. Maybe some of them will answer some

211

questions you have about your own sciatica. Be sure to remember the caution at the front of the book. Nothing here is designed to be a substitute for your visit to your own doctor. All we're trying to do is to give you some information you can use in conjunction with what your doctor, therapist or practitioner tells you.

Q. If I sit all day on my thick wallet, can that have any effect on my back and my sciatica?

A. It certainly can. By sitting on your wallet it can throw your balance off and you'll be compensating for the tilt to one side or the other. This can put an unneeded strain on your back and could even help to bring on a sciatica attack. Most pants are made so the wallet is not that far under the buttocks. The wallet can be more to the side. If your pants are not constructed that way, carry your wallet in your jacket pocket. You might also want to check on pockets when you buy new pants.

Q. Why aren't homeopathic medications under the control of the Food And Drug Administration?

A. Back in 1938 the law was written so the medicines listed in the homeopathic pharmacopoeia of medications were exempt from many of the FDA controls. Why? Because the substances

212

were investigated by the writers of the law and they discovered that the chemical elements in these prescriptions were so diluted that they could not be harmful. A homeopathic medication that contains arsenic, for example, contains such a minute quantify of arsenic, that a child could eat a whole bottle full and suffer no harmful effects. However, if broad or vague claims are made for cures of diseases, the FDA will step in and take control.

Q. Why is my grandmother now shorter than she was when she was a young woman?

A. There are thirty-two discs between your vertebrae. These pillows or shock absorbers are usually somewhere around three-sixteenths of an inch thick. As a person gets older, there is a gradual wearing away and compressing of these discs. By the age of sixty, many individuals have lost as much as one-eighth of an inch from each of those pads. That times thirty two means that your grandmother could well be four inches shorter now at seventy years than she was when she was thirty. Some doctors refer to this as degenerative changes. Usually this doesn't cause a lot of trouble, unless the disc vanishes altogether and the vertebrae start grinding against each other.

Q. Can large breasts contribute to back

pain?

A. Yes. Excessively large breasts can cause several problems beside wolf whistles. These include headaches, neck strain, low back pain, aching shoulders and even tingling in the fingers. The added weight of large breasts can shift a woman's center of gravity forward which put a big strain on the low back muscles and puts more pressure on the lower and upper back. Many times women with large breasts will try to diminish their appearance by rolling their shoulders forward and in and even rounding the spine. All this does is de-emphasize the breasts slightly but puts a huge pressure on the back again. Many women with this condition investigate breast reduction to help solve the back and other problems. Talk with your doctor and with a plastic surgeon to find out if this procedure will help you.

Q. I've heard about CAT scans and a CT scan. What's the difference? Which one is best?

A. No difference. CAT and CT are simply two different terms for the same thing. Most civilians probably use CAT scan, while many doctors and nurses say CT scan. The initials stand for Computerized Axial Tomography. That simply means it's a diagnostic form of radiology. It is becoming more and more common and in back problem cases can be used to find a herniated or prolapsed disc that an X-ray can't see. The X-ray shows only bones, while the CAT scan can give a good rendering of soft tissue such as the discs between your vertebrae.

The CAT scan takes about twenty minutes to picture your spine. It is used many times in place of a myelogram and is less invasive and less painful.

Q. My father had two herniated discs and they fused his spine. He was miserable for the last ten years of his life. Does this mean that I'll have herniated discs as well?

A. There is no firm evidence that this is true. Many discs herniate because of the activity of the patient not from some hereditary precondition. If you do the same construction work your father did, you have a chance of getting the same problem. If he was in construction but the heaviest thing you lift is a mouse on your computer, you just might never have a ruptured disc.

Q. I'm getting over a herniated disc. Does this mean that I might get another one soon?

A. Yes and no. If you are working at the same job, lifting the same loads, behaving in the same way physically that you did just before you herniated the disc the first time, it well could happen

215

again in the same disc or in another one nearby. To prevent this, take better care of your back, reduce the risk of injury to your back, practice good posture and take all precautions practical against irritating and damaging your spinal column.

Q. I have a backache. Should I go directly to a specialist?

A. No. It's usually best to go to your GP or family doctor first and tell him your troubles and what hurts. This first doctor will do a preliminary examination, ask you a lot of questions, have you do some exercises that can pinpoint certain back problems. If he thinks you need to see an expert on the spine, he will send you along. If your problem is minor and one that he can help you with, you'll find relief with him.

Q. What's an osteopath? I've never heard of one.

A. The term is better known in some states than in others. In some states the osteopath physician is on an equal footing with an M.D. They work in the same clinics and hospitals, have the same public respect, treat the same diseases and conditions. Both can prescribe medications and do surgery. The osteopath is more likely to try non-surgical methods where possible and may not rely on medications as much as an M.D.

In some states the Osteopath is a "second

class" doctor and can't work in M.D. hospitals. This is by state licensing practices. In those states the osteopaths have their own hospitals, agencies and organizations.

Q. My friend says chiropractors are great healers, but some just have a bad name. Is that true?

A. In the chiropractic field there is a wide range of skilled people. They range all the way from fine healers, to the fair and then to the bad and the careless and the out and out charlatans. Many chiropractors will try to set you up with a structured program of eight, ten, twelve even twenty-four visits to take care of a problem. If you want to go to a chiropractor, check carefully into his or her qualifications, talk to patients, and know exactly what care you want from the chiropractor. As a gentle reminder, for any ailment, it's usually good to go to your family M.D. first. He or she has better training to do a complete diagnosis of any problem you may have.

Q. If ninety percent of back problems go away in two months, why should I go to a doctor at all?

A. True, most back pains will either go away or become much less severe in sixty days as the body works at healing itself. However, those sixty days can be pure hell in many cases. The doctor

217

visit will help you to deal with the pain through medications or physical therapy or other suggestions. Also, if you are one of those ten percent who has a herniated disc that must be treated, it's better to know about it right away, rather than waiting out the two months of pain, only to find out you're one of the unlucky ten percent.

Q. What's the bottom line on faith healers, herbalists, homeopaths, acupuncturists, reflexologists and acupressurists who say they can help heal my aching sciatica?

A. Remember the sixty day healing or "living with" self healing mentioned above. So say you've worried your aching back with ibuprofen and naproxen sodium for six weeks and your back is still furious and hurting like hell. You decide to go to a reflexologist and after two weeks of treatments, your back is much better. Hey, you can say the reflexologist really cured you, or you can know that after the sixty days you would have been a lot better anyway. Part of this back healing is simply common sense.

The bottom line is that sometimes the fringe elements of medicine can really help, sometimes they don't help, sometimes people who wish for help hard enough get it from psychosomatic input. Take your choice and take your chances.

Q. I've heard of a bone scan in conjunction with sciatica. What is a bone scan? It sounds scary.

A. A bone scan is a type of X-ray that gives you little radiation exposure. A drawback is that it takes four hours to complete. During a bone scan you'll need to lie face down on a table for a whole hour. A bone scan will show healed fractures, tumors and infections and arthritis in the joints and bones of your spine. Routine X-rays of your low back give you ten times as much radiation exposure as a bone scan.

Q. What's an MRI? I hear one can cost $4,000. Is this true?

A. The letters MRI stand for Magnetic Resonance Imaging. It is not an X-ray. It uses magnetic fields and radio waves. It can give doctors pictures of the spine or other parts of the body from different angles and views. It can show plainly if a disc is herniated. It will show up problems with the spine, tumors or other ailments and even give evidence of diseased tissue. Costs vary according to the length of time needed to do the MRI scan. Some costs can be as much as $4,000, but most are much less.

Q. How soon can I get back to work after a bad sciatica attack?

A. That depends on a lot of factors. Primary

is what work are you doing? If you're laying eighteen pound concrete blocks and mortaring them into a wall twenty feet high and working on a scaffold, you won't be back at work for a month, maybe two. If you are a file clerk or a waitress or a store clerk, you might get back on the job two weeks after your pain is manageable. It depends on your job, your ability to work over a little bit of pain, and how much you need that paycheck.

Q. Is it true that an acupressurist is only an acupuncturist who uses his thumbs and fingers instead of needles on the same pressure points?

A. Some people will say yes. Some no. Basically the two systems seem to be remarkably similar using the same body areas and pressure or needles with electrical input to establish the same overload on major nerves. How close together they are is up for speculation. Number wise there are many more with the needles than without.

Q. If I wear high heeled shoes, will it hurt my back?

A. If you wear five or six inch spikes, it's going to be bad for your back as long as you're standing or walking. The heels throw the entire body out of balance and the tendency is to effect a swayback position with all of the dangers and problems.

If you stick to two inch heels, there is far less chance that the swayback problem will come up. Even two inch heels can cause you some backache. If it doesn't, feel free to wear the low heels. If you need two inch heels, try to wear them for as short a period as possible. A spare pair of shoes at the office with lower heels or even flats is a good plan. Also a good pair of sneakers for that walk to the subway or to your parking lot is always a healthy choice.

Q. I heard my doctor talking about the two year sciatic rule. What is that?

A. There is a general opinion among doctors specializing in back problems that most patients who have sciatica attacks will have another one within two years. The figure is about sixty percent. That's probably for those who don't take better care of their backs after the first attack. You won't make that mistake so you can keep in that sciatic attack free forty percent. Good back care and exercises to strengthen back muscles will help you to prevent a second sciatic attack.

Q. Why did my doctor tell me to quit the stretching exercises I was doing? I thought it was good for my back.

A. Probably it would be good for a well back. If you have back pain or sciatica, some of the stretches actually stretch the sciatic nerve and this

221

increases your problem and your pain. This usually happens with those who have had recent sciatic problems. Stretching exercises are used to loosen up the ligaments in the back area of the spine and tight hamstrings. Usually they're good. If they hurt, don't do them.

Q. I heard people with backaches used to use gravity boots. What ever happened to them?

A. With gravity boots the idea is to hang upside down. This can be done a variety of ways. Some experts like the idea. Others say that it can cause a few other problems not related to stretching out your spine. Some are: increase in blood pressure and heart rate. Nerves in your ankles can show irritation and with prolonged upside down hanging, you could suffer bleeding in the back of the eye. On balance, forget about the upside down hang.

Q. How much of the disc is removed in surgery?

A. Usually only the herniated part and maybe twenty percent of the soft matter in the center of the disc. All loose material is removed. Almost never is the whole disc removed. That would leave nothing to separate the vertebrae and you'd be in bigger trouble than ever. Usually there is enough of the disc and soft core left to do the shock absorbing job the disc was designed to do.

Q. My friend with sciatica said he didn't try to have sex for six months after his back felt better. Isn't that too long to wait?

A. Sexual intercourse can and should be undertaken as soon as the person feels ready. If the sciatic pain is mostly gone, try the spoon position described in a previous chapter. Be careful not to bend your back, always bend your hips. If your first attempt causes too much pain, wait a while. Six months is way too long.

Q. I'm having a discotomy. Can I give my blood for use during my surgery?

A. Almost always. Most hospitals will draw your blood before surgery and hold it for use when you go in the operating room. Check with your hospital for their time frames and schedules and about costs. Most people feel more secure using their own blood if any is required during surgery. Find out how many pints are usually needed and plan ahead.

Q. I like to sleep on my stomach, but my wife says that's hard on my back. Is she right?

A. You lose, depending how you sleep. If you use pillows in the right places, you can still sleep on your stomach. Use a pillow for your head that will keep your head in a straight line with your back, not pushed up or dropped down. Then

223

support your stomach with a pillow or a lumbar roll. Fasten this around your waist so it will support your stomach or your back if you turn over during the night.

Q. Why is it better to push a heavy object than to pull it?

A. When you push a couch or a big box, you can dig in your feet and use your body weight as well as the thrust of your muscles to push an item. On the other hand when you try to pull something, you have only your muscles to do the job. You're short half of your resources. So always push, instead of pull.

Q. Is hypnosis pure quackery or is there some value?

A. Many people use hypnosis to alter their state of mind with the hope that this will help alter their physical side. For some, it works, for others it is not quite right. Learn as much as you can about hypnotism, then go to a registered hypnotist and have that person hypnotize you. Get the feel of it. If you like it, get training so you can hypnotize yourself. Hypnotism might not cure your sciatic back, but for some people it can help them to endure the pain and to take a different approach to it.

Q. After an injury or pain, is it ice first or heat first?

A. Watch pro football. The ice pack comes on the moment an injured player hits the sidelines. Ice tends to reduce swelling and to downgrade pain. The use of heat comes a day later to bring fresh blood to the injured area to speed the recovery. After the first day some people think that alternating heat and ice packs helps speed recovery.

Q. **How can I get Tylenol-4? I hear that it is a wonderful pain killer.**

A. The only way to get Tylenol-4 is with a prescription. This medication contains the largest amount of codeine in any prescription drug and most doctors are cautious about prescribing it. Codeine is a highly addictive drug. Tylenol-4 would be used only for the most debilitating pain. A sciatic attack usually would not qualify by most doctors for the strong pain killer.

Q. **Whatever happened to that month long bed rest plan after a sciatica attack?**

A. It went out with the polyester suit. Times change, we learn. The long term bed rest was finally determined to cause more problems than the good it did. The back is a functional mechanism. It isn't functioning when lying in bed. Normal use of the spine, after a day or two of bed rest, turned out to be the best for the patient. Problems such as bed sores, a deterioration of

225

muscles for walking and sitting up all led to the cutting bed rest from thirty days to two by most doctors.

Q. I saw a headline about a $300 injection that can do the job of a $10,000 back surgery. What does that mean?

A. That is chymopapain, a substance that is injected into the disc that "melts down" the soft core of the disc that has prolapsed or herniated and is pressing against the sciatic nerve root causing the pain. When the material there melts from the shot, it is carried away by the blood and eventually discharged from the body in urine. This does the same thing a discotomy does, except it is done simply, is less intrusive, creates no blood loss or healing of surgical procedures, and costs only about $300. A discotomy with doctors and operating room and all usually costs about $10,000. Many doctors are now looking at the injection as a good substitute for the discotomy. It is much easier on the patient, from a pain and suffering, recovery and a financial basis.

Q. Does a bulging disc always mean the person has back pain?

A. No. Recent studies show that with MRI and CAT Scan, many patients are found to have herniated discs and bulging discs, yet they have no back pain. In persons over forty, it was found that fifty percent of them had bulging discs but no pain. In another study thirty five percent of persons checked who were over forty had herniated discs yet no pain. Here the spinal canal was probably large enough to allow for the herniation or bulging so it did not press hard on the root nerve to cause any pain.

Q. **With all this talk about the back and the spine, isn't it a rather delicate structure we should treat with care?**

A. Not at all. Actually the spine is a finely built foundation for the back that can take a lot of pressure, and withstand tremendous forces without injury. The secret is to be sure that the muscles that support the back are kept strong with good flexibility and endurance. These are maintained with the correct body mechanics and good posture.

Q. **Is it true that it puts more strain on your back to sit than it does to stand? How can that be?**

A. Yes, true. Standing is easier on your back. It's the mechanics of the thing. By sitting there is more weight concentrated on the lower back than when standing. It's a matter of weight and muscle use and tension and all that sort of scientific stuff. Believe sitting is harder on a back, especially if it's hurting.

Q. I've heard that the older a person gets, the worse the back becomes and more pain and misery. Is this right?

A. You heard it wrong. The fact is that back pain and problems peak in the thirty-five to fifty-five years of your life. After that back pain and problems actually decreases for most people. Now the spine will continue to degenerate as the discs shrink and wear away. That's why older people get shorter. But as far as backs and the spine problems getting worse and worse in the sixties, seventies and eighties, it just isn't so.

Q. A friend told me that because of my back pain, I should go to his doctor because he started out with an X-ray of the spine and back to be sure everything was right. Is this the usual procedure?

A. No. Most doctors go through their regular diagnosis procedure for patients with back pain to try to tie down the cause and the problem. This usually is after two or three weeks of conservative treatment of two days of rest, then medications, and other conservative methods. If these do not solve the problem or show the cause, then the X-ray is usually used. These days the X-ray might not be used and a CAT scan given instead since it's a better diagnostic tool in many ways.

228

Q. Why would a doctor use psychological testing when working on a diagnosis for back pain? Seems weird.

A. Some doctors find a need for psychological testing if the patient does not respond to other methods. Psychological testing can be used for several reasons. Among them: if the patient has serious depression or anxiety, if there is substance abuse such as alcohol, drugs or addiction to prescription drugs, lack of the ability to cope with pain, or it's suspected the pain may be partly stress related. Not weird at all.

Q. What good is ultrasound in back treatment?

A. Ultrasound does much the same thing as moist heat. It warms the tissue and simply reduces some pain and makes you feel better. Ultrasound is the use of sound waves with a higher frequency than the human ear can hear. The ultrasound waves as used here are absorbed by the tissue warming it and reducing the pain. This is not a treatment to cure the problem. When ultrasound is used it is to provide short term relief from the pain, similar to that offered by moist heat.

Q. What is chronic opioid therapy as used for back pain?

A. It's a controversial treatment not much

used in the United States. Simply put it's the long term use of highly addictive drugs such as opiates and morphine to control a patient's pain. Most doctors won't even consider such drastic medication because of the high incidence of addiction as well as the side effects and the patient's tolerance for the drugs. Side effects include serious constipation, insomnia, decreased sexual function, trouble thinking and focusing.

Q. Is the antidepressant Prozac used much for back pain?

A. Sometimes. Prozac is one of six or eight antidepressants that some doctors feel has some beneficial effect in some patients when they have depression and back pain. One of the reasons to use an antidepressant would be when a back patient has serious problems sleeping. Some of the antidepressant drugs will help normalize sleeping and also help reduce the pain associated with the back problems. The use of drugs such as Prozac would be in extreme cases only and for a limited time.

Q. Is it true that sitting too long on a toilet seat can irritate an already screaming sciatic nerve?

A. Absolutely true. Also too much straining to have a bowel movement can do the same thing. If you have or are getting over a sciatic attack here are some other ways you can strain and irritate that already hurting sciatic nerve: Don't sit on cold concrete for any length of time. Don't over-stretch before exercising, take it easy. Low, underslung car seats can irritate your sciatic nerve. Too little flesh on your bottom can irritate the sciatic nerve if you do a lot of sitting. Try a good soft pillow. Even a lumpy, uneven pillow can irritate your already sensitive sciatic nerve.

Q. Is it just an old wives' tale that hot baths will help a hurting back and sciatic problems?

A. Not at all. A good warm bath for twenty minutes will do wonders for that hurting back. Why? The warm infusion in the body reduces stiffness in the muscles and joints and brings a rush of new blood through the affected areas. The warmth opens the blood vessels more than usual so more blood gets to muscles and into the tissue.

For another aid, try putting a double handful of Epsom salts into your warm bath. This is magnesium sulfate and it opens your pores and induces perspiration. This helps cleans your body inside.

After twenty minutes let the Epsom salts water out and rinse off with fresh warm water from the tap. This will close up your pores and

231

get your circulation back in balance. Then get out of the tub slowly so you don't pass out. You may get a little light headed but it will pass.

Q. My shoulder purse gets heavy sometimes when it looks more like a suitcase. Can this hurt my sore back?

A. You bet it can hurt. Dump out your purse and leave at home everything you don't absolutely need to take with you. Try using one of your smaller purses so you can't overload it. Be sure to shift even a shoulder strap purse from side to side during the day. If you have lots to carry, do it with a backpack instead of a briefcase. Might not be as fashionable, but it's much easier on your back, and they might think you're still in school.

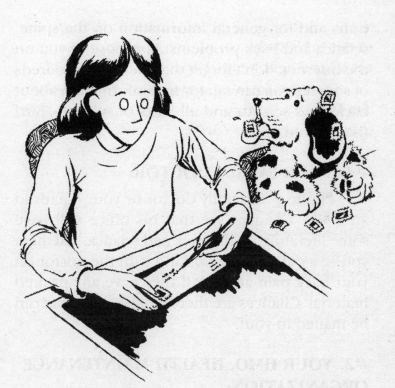

CHAPTER THIRTEEN:
INFORMATION SOURCES FOR BACK PAIN

There is a wealth of information available these days on almost any topic you care to research—including sciatica and back pain. Give these sources a whirl to get specific answers to questions and for general information on the spine, sciatica and back problems. For those of you on the Internet, don't forget that there are hundreds of sources you can tap for free information about backs and sciatica and all sorts of subjects. Surf the net and see.

#1. YOUR FAMILY DOCTOR:

Phone your family doctor or your doctor in an HMO. Chances are that his office will have some literature on the back and sciatica. Tell them you're a patient and working with the doctor on your back pain and ask if they have any printed material. Chances are there will be some that can be mailed to you.

#2. YOUR HMO, HEALTH MAINTENANCE ORGANIZATION:

If you are a member of a large HMO, such as Kaiser, your local HMO hospital probably has a library. Call them and ask them what they have on sciatica and back problems. They may be able to mail you material, or invite you down to read their reference material in the library. Many of these are quite helpful.

234

#3. THE U.S. GOVERNMENT:

Yes, true. There is a U.S. government service that the federal government operates that will give you information on any health problem. It may be in the form of literature or they may give you referrals to libraries or organizations. The toll free number is:

800-336-4797

#4: INTERNATIONAL COLLEGE OF ACUPUNCTURE:

800 Riverside Drive #8-1
New York, NY 10032

This is a nonprofit educational organization that is chartered by the University of the State of New York. It promotes research and teaching of safe and effective acupuncture and related treatments including herbal medicine. It works to combine the best of Western and Oriental medicine through international cooperation and shares its findings with the public.

5: ALLIANCE FOUNDATION FOR ALTERNATIVE MEDICINE

P.O. Box 59
Liberty Lake, WA 99019
509-255-9246

235

This foundation offers current research material on alternative health care and prevention of disease. It publishes a number of reports and books on alternative health care practices.

#6: HEALTH WORLD:

> 1477 Rollins Road
> Burlingame, CA 94010
> 415-343-1637

Publishes a wide variety of health information on vitamins, nutrition, homeopathy and Chinese medicine.

#7: JOURNAL OF ALTERNATIVE AND COMPLEMENTARY MEDICINE:

> Manner House
> 53A High Street
> Bag Shot. Surrey
> GUl95AH
> England

In Europe, herbal preparations outsell over-the-counter drugs. Many Americans are surprised to learn this. As a general rule, there are only a few sources of information on alternative remedies available to Americans in the U.S. This organization publishes a monthly newsletter devoted to alternative and complementary medicine.

236

#8: NATIONAL ASSOCIATION FOR HOLISTIC AROMATHERAPY:

P.O. Box 17622
Boulder, Colorado 80308
303-258-3791

This group publishes a newsletter on aromatherapy. More than sixty aromatic substances exhibit healing properties. When applied to the skin, these substances can aid healing. When they are inhaled, it is said that they trigger a reaction in the brain which can achieve therapeutic effects.

#9: ASSOCIATION FOR APPLIED PSYCHOPHYSIOLOGY & BIOFEEDBACK:

10200 West 44th Ave #304
Wheat Ridge, CO 80033
300-422-8436

The association pursues continuing study in biofeedback. It has over two thousand members around the U.S. It can provide referrals for you to locate qualified professionals in your area.

#10: ALLERGY ALERT:

P.O. Box 31065
Seattle, WA 98103
206-547-1814

237

Issues a self help newsletter on the latest food allergies research, cooking tips and proper diet information

#11: FOOD ALLERGY CENTER:

> 53-31 Marathon Parkway
> Little Neck, NY 11362
> l-800-YES-RELIEF

The center is a resource for general information about food allergies and sensitivities. Information is provided on the various alternative treatments available. A newsletter is also published.

#12: ASSOCIATION OF HOLISTIC HEALING CENTERS:

> 2100 Mediterranean Avenue #40
> Virginia Beach, VA 23451
> 804-498-2598

The association offers holistic healing practitioners referral information and further information on the healing arts.

#13: AMERICAN BOTANICAL COUNCIL:

> P.O. Box 201660
> Austin, TX 78720
> 512-331-8868

The council conducts research and education supporting herb folk remedies, teas and other herb based products. It also publishes a quarterly newsletter.

#14: AMERICAN HERB ASSOCIATION:

P.O. Box 353
Rescue, CA 95672
916-626-5046

This organization provides up to date research on herbal health, herb gardening and new herbal products. The association also publishes several herbal source directories.

#15: INTERNATIONAL FOUNDATION FOR HOMEOPATHY:

2366 Eastlake Avenue East #301
Seattle, WA 98102
206-234-8230

The foundation promotes homeopathic science through education, training and public relations. As an information clearing house, the foundation answers questions on homeopathy and provides referrals to homeopathic practitioners in your area.

#16: ACADEMY OF SCIENTIFIC HYPNOTHERAPY:

P.O. Box 12041
San Diego, CA 92112
619-427-6255

The academy acts as a clearinghouse for information and makes referrals to local hypnotherapists in your area.

#17: THE NATIONAL SOCIETY OF HYPNOTHERAPISTS:

2175 NW 85th #6A
Des Moines, IA 50325
515-270-2280

This group publishes a quarterly newsletter on new developments in hypnotherapy and makes referrals to qualified hypnotherapists in your area.

#18: AMERICAN ASSOCIATION OF NATUROPATHIC PHYSICIANS:

2800 East Madison Street #200
Seattle, WA 98112
206-323-7610

Naturopaths are trained as specialists in the use of natural therapeutics and restoring overall health. Where required, they must pass a state licensing examination.

240

#19: AMERICAN BOARD OF NUTRITION:

9650 Rockville Pike
Bethesda, MD 20814
301-530-7110

This board helps establish standards and certifies those who are able to pass an examination. The board can provide a list of qualified professional nutritionists in your area.

#20: AMERICAN NUTRITIONISTS' ASSOCIATION:

5530 Wisconsin Avenue NW #1149
Washington, DC 20815
301-657-4751

This is a professional organization of nutritionists, most of whom have advanced degrees. The association promotes education and publishes a quarterly newsletter.

#21: THE PRESIDENT'S COUNCIL ON FITNESS:

Department of Health,
Education & Welfare
Room 3030 Donohoe Bldg.
400 Sixth St. S. W.
Washington, DC 20201
202-755-7947

For information about exercising and physical fitness.

#22: NATIONAL INSTITUTE OF MENTAL HEALTH:

Room 11A33, Parklawn Bldg.
5600 Fishers Lane
Rockville, Maryland 20857
301-443-4517

For stress control information.

#23: THE NATIONAL COUNCIL ON ALCOHOLISM:

733 Third Avenue
New York, NY 10017
212-986-4433

For help with any kind of alcohol addition, aid, referrals, local organizations, information, literature.

APPENDIX:
EXERCISE AND AEROBIC CHARTS FOR YOUR RECORDKEEPING

On the following twelve pages you'll find charts, one for every day of the next year, so you can chart out your daily exercise and/or aerobic activity. The key at the bottom shows your level of work. They go from level one through ten showing how many repetitions you do on each one. Enjoy.

243

		EXERCISE #																					LEVEL ___		AEROBICS		
Date	Warm	1	2	3	4	5	6	7	8	9	10	11	12	13	14	15	16	17	18	19	20	21	22	23	24	Cool	Type	Time	Weight
1																													
2																													
3																													
4																													
5																													
6																													
7																													
8																													
9																													
10																													
11																													
12																													
13																													
14																													
15																													
16																													
17																													
18																													
19																													
20																													
21																													
22																													
23																													
24																													
25																													
26																													
27																													
28																													
29																													
30																													
31																													

244

Development Levels: #1-4 reps, #2-6 reps, #3- 8 resp, #4-10 reps, #5-12 reps, #6-16 reps, #7-18 reps, #8-20 reps, #9-22 reps, #10-24 reps

EXERCISE #   LEVEL____   AEROBICS

Date	Warm	1	2	3	4	5	6	7	8	9	10	11	12	13	14	15	16	17	18	19	20	21	22	23	24	Cool	Type	Time	Weight
1																													
2																													
3																													
4																													
5																													
6																													
7																													
8																													
9																													
10																													
11																													
12																													
13																													
14																													
15																													
16																													
17																													
18																													
19																													
20																													
21																													
22																													
23																													
24																													
25																													
26																													
27																													
28																													
29																													
30																													
31																													

245

Development Levels: #1-4 reps, #2-6 reps, #3- 8 resp, #4-10 reps, #5-12 reps, #6-16 reps, #7-18 reps, #8-20 reps, #9-22 reps, #10-24 reps

EXERCISE #   LEVEL _____

																										AEROBICS		
Date	Warm	1	2	3	4	5	6	7	8	9	10	11	12	13	14	15	16	17	18	19	20	21	22	23	24	Cool	Type	Time	Weight
1																													
2																													
3																													
4																													
5																													
6																													
7																													
8																													
9																													
10																													
11																													
12																													
13																													
14																													
15																													
16																													
17																													
18																													
19																													
20																													
21																													
22																													
23																													
24																													
25																													
26																													
27																													
28																													
29																													
30																													
31																													

Development Levels: #1-4 reps, #2-6 reps, #3- 8 resp, #4-10 reps, #5-12 reps, #6-16 reps, #7-18 reps, #8-20 reps, #9-22 reps, #10-24 reps

EXERCISE #   LEVEL ___   AEROBICS

Date	Warm	1	2	3	4	5	6	7	8	9	10	11	12	13	14	15	16	17	18	19	20	21	22	23	24	Cool	Type	Time	Weight
1																													
2																													
3																													
4																													
5																													
6																													
7																													
8																													
9																													
10																													
11																													
12																													
13																													
14																													
15																													
16																													
17																													
18																													
19																													
20																													
21																													
22																													
23																													
24																													
25																													
26																													
27																													
28																													
29																													
30																													
31																													

247

Development Levels: #1-4 reps, #2-6 reps, #3- 8 resp, #4-10 reps, #5-12 reps, #6-16 reps, #7-18 reps, #8-20 reps, #9-22 reps, #10-24 reps

		EXERCISE #											LEVEL___													AEROBICS			
Date	Warm	1	2	3	4	5	6	7	8	9	10	11	12	13	14	15	16	17	18	19	20	21	22	23	24	Cool	Type	Time	Weight
1																													
2																													
3																													
4																													
5																													
6																													
7																													
8																													
9																													
10																													
11																													
12																													
13																													
14																													
15																													
16																													
17																													
18																													
19																													
20																													
21																													
22																													
23																													
24																													
25																													
26																													
27																													
28																													
29																													
30																													
31																													

248

Development Levels: #1-4 reps, #2-6 reps, #3- 8 resp, #4-10 reps, #5-12 reps, #6-16 reps, #7-18 reps, #8-20 reps, #9-22 reps, #10-24 reps

EXERCISE #   LEVEL _____

																										AEROBICS		
Date	Warm	1	2	3	4	5	6	7	8	9	10	11	12	13	14	15	16	17	18	19	20	21	22	23	24	Cool	Type	Time	Weight
1																													
2																													
3																													
4																													
5																													
6																													
7																													
8																													
9																													
10																													
11																													
12																													
13																													
14																													
15																													
16																													
17																													
18																													
19																													
20																													
21																													
22																													
23																													
24																													
25																													
26																													
27																													
28																													
29																													
30																													
31																													

Development Levels: #1-4 reps, #2-6 reps, #3- 8 resp, #4-10 reps, #5-12 reps, #6-16 reps, #7-18 reps, #8-20 reps, #9-22 reps, #10-24 reps

249

EXERCISE #   LEVEL _____

Date	Warm	1	2	3	4	5	6	7	8	9	10	11	12	13	14	15	16	17	18	19	20	21	22	23	24	Cool	AEROBICS Type	Time	Weight
1																													
2																													
3																													
4																													
5																													
6																													
7																													
8																													
9																													
10																													
11																													
12																													
13																													
14																													
15																													
16																													
17																													
18																													
19																													
20																													
21																													
22																													
23																													
24																													
25																													
26																													
27																													
28																													
29																													
30																													
31																													

Development Levels: #1-4 reps, #2-6 reps, #3- 8 resp, #4-10 reps, #5-12 reps, #6-16 reps, #7-18 reps, #8-20 reps, #9-22 reps, #10-24 reps

EXERCISE #   LEVEL ___   AEROBICS

Date	Warm	1	2	3	4	5	6	7	8	9	10	11	12	13	14	15	16	17	18	19	20	21	22	23	24	Cool	Type	Time	Weight
1																													
2																													
3																													
4																													
5																													
6																													
7																													
8																													
9																													
10																													
11																													
12																													
13																													
14																													
15																													
16																													
17																													
18																													
19																													
20																													
21																													
22																													
23																													
24																													
25																													
26																													
27																													
28																													
29																													
30																													
31																													

Development Levels: #1-4 reps, #2-6 reps, #3- 8 resp, #4-10 reps, #5-12 reps, #6-16 reps, #7-18 reps, #8-20 reps, #9-22 reps, #10-24 reps

		EXERCISE #																							LEVEL___		AEROBICS		
Date	Warm	1	2	3	4	5	6	7	8	9	10	11	12	13	14	15	16	17	18	19	20	21	22	23	24	Cool	Type	Time	Weight
1																													
2																													
3																													
4																													
5																													
6																													
7																													
8																													
9																													
10																													
11																													
12																													
13																													
14																													
15																													
16																													
17																													
18																													
19																													
20																													
21																													
22																													
23																													
24																													
25																													
26																													
27																													
28																													
29																													
30																													
31																													

Development Levels: #1-4 reps, #2-6 reps, #3- 8 resp, #4-10 reps, #5-12 reps, #6-16 reps, #7-18 reps, #8-20 reps, #9-22 reps, #10-24 reps

AEROBICS

Date	Warm	1	2	3	4	5	6	7	8	9	10	11	12	13	14	15	16	17	18	19	20	21	22	23	24	Cool	Type	Time	Weight
1																													
2																													
3																													
4																													
5																													
6																													
7																													
8																													
9																													
10																													
11																													
12																													
13																													
14																													
15																													
16																													
17																													
18																													
19																													
20																													
21																													
22																													
23																													
24																													
25																													
26																													
27																													
28																													
29																													
30																													
31																													

Development Levels: #1-4 reps, #2-6 reps, #3- 8 resp, #4-10 reps, #5-12 reps, #6-16 reps, #7-18 reps, #8-20 reps, #9-22 reps, #10-24 reps

EXERCISE #   LEVEL ___   AEROBICS

Date	Warm	1	2	3	4	5	6	7	8	9	10	11	12	13	14	15	16	17	18	19	20	21	22	23	24	Cool	Type	Time	Weight
1																													
2																													
3																													
4																													
5																													
6																													
7																													
8																													
9																													
10																													
11																													
12																													
13																													
14																													
15																													
16																													
17																													
18																													
19																													
20																													
21																													
22																													
23																													
24																													
25																													
26																													
27																													
28																													
29																													
30																													
31																													

Development Levels: #1-4 reps, #2-6 reps, #3- 8 resp, #4-10 reps, #5-12 reps, #6-16 reps, #7-18 reps, #8-20 reps, #9-22 reps, #10-24 reps

EXERCISE #   LEVEL ___   AEROBICS

Date	Warm	1	2	3	4	5	6	7	8	9	10	11	12	13	14	15	16	17	18	19	20	21	22	23	24	Cool	Type	Time	Weight
1																													
2																													
3																													
4																													
5																													
6																													
7																													
8																													
9																													
10																													
11																													
12																													
13																													
14																													
15																													
16																													
17																													
18																													
19																													
20																													
21																													
22																													
23																													
24																													
25																													
26																													
27																													
28																													
29																													
30																													
31																													

Development Levels: #1-4 reps, #2-6 reps, #3- 8 resp, #4-10 reps, #5-12 reps, #6-16 reps, #7-18 reps, #8-20 reps, #9-22 reps, #10-24 reps

255

NOTES

INDEX

A

Acupuncture *61, 62, 63, 65, 69, 117, 118, 235*
Addiction *43, 229, 230*
Analgesic *40, 114*
Anesthetic *49, 108*
Ankylosing spondyltis *18, 19*
Annulus *33*
Anti-inflammatory *40, 114*
Antidepressant *230*
Arthritis *18, 19, 20, 24, 79, 219*

B

Back pain *19, 21, 22, 41, 42, 45, 48, 55, 57, 60, 67, 73, 76, 77, 78, 82, 83, 86, 97, 101, 102, 103, 104, 111, 112, 119, 124, 130, 131, 163, 187, 190, 193, 195, 198, 201, 208, 209, 213, 214, 217, 221, 226, 228, 229, 230, 233, 234*
Biofeedback *59, 118, 126, 237*
Bone scan *219*
Bone spurs *20*
Bulging disc *15, 17, 18, 21, 103, 226, 227*

C

CAT scan *24, 25, 26, 27, 102, 107, 214, 215, 226, 228*
Center of gravity *206, 214*

Sciatica Relief Handbook

Stress *12, 17, 21, 23, 53, 56, 59, 69, 83, 118, 122,
123, 124, 125, 126, 127, 140, 160, 161, 162,
169, 171, 177, 182, 185, 194, 201, 205, 207,
229, 242*
Symptom *21, 28, 53, 57, 77, 89, 90, 91, 92, 125*

T

Tendon *95, 96*
TENS *47, 48*
Thoracic *30, 35*
Tolerance *230*
Traction *47, 74, 94, 96, 194*
Trigger point *48, 68*

U

Ultrasound *49, 73, 74, 229*

V

Vertebra *11, 12, 14, 19, 20, 21, 24, 25, 28, 31, 32,
34, 35, 36, 37, 64, 67, 68, 78, 102, 103, 104,
105, 201, 207, 213, 215, 222*

X

X-Ray *24, 26, 27, 28, 72, 75, 79, 93, 95, 104, 105,
109, 208, 215, 219, 228*

NOTES